Current Topics in Transplantation

Editor

A. OSAMA GABER

SURGICAL CLINICS OF NORTH AMERICA

www.surgical.theclinics.com

Consulting Editor
RONALD F. MARTIN

December 2013 • Volume 93 • Number 6

ELSEVIER

1600 John F. Kennedy Boulevard ● Suite 1800 ● Philadelphia, Pennsylvania, 19103-2899

http://www.surgical.theclinics.com

SURGICAL CLINICS OF NORTH AMERICA Volume 93, Number 6
December 2013 ISSN 0039–6109, ISBN-13: 978-0-323-26130-2

Editor: John Vassallo, j.vassallo@elsevier.com
Developmental Editor: Yonah Korngold

Surgical Clinics of North America (ISSN 0039–6109) is published bimonthly by Elsevier Inc., 360 Park Avenue South, New York, NY 10010-1710. Months of publication are February, April, June, August, October, and December. Business and Editorial Offices: 1600 John F. Kennedy Blvd., Suite 1800, Philadelphia, PA 19103-2899. Periodicals postage paid at New York, NY and additional mailing offices. Subscription prices are $370.00 per year for US individuals, $627.00 per year for US institutions, $180.00 per year for US students and residents, $455.00 per year for Canadian individuals, $793.00 per year for Canadian institutions, $510.00 for international individuals, $793.00 per year for international institutions and $250.00 per year for Canadian and foreign students/residents. To receive student/resident rate, orders must be accompanied by name of affiliated institution, date of term, and the *signature* of program/residency coordinator on institution letterhead. Orders will be billed at individual rate until proof of status is received. Foreign air speed delivery is included in all *Clinics* subscription prices. All prices are subject to change without notice. POSTMASTER: Send address changes to *Surgical Clinics*, Elsevier Health Sciences Division, Subscription Customer Service, 3251 Riverport Lane, Maryland Heights, MO 63043. **Customer Service (orders, claims, online, change of address): Telephone: 1-800-654-2452 (U.S. and Canada); 314-447-8871 (outside U.S. and Canada). Fax: 314-447-8029. E-mail: journalscustomerservice-usa@elsevier.com (for print support); journalsonline support-usa@elsevier.com (for online support).**

Reprints. For copies of 100 or more, of articles in this publication, please contact the Commercial Reprints Department, Elsevier Inc., 360 Park Avenue South, New York, New York 10010-1710. Tel. 212-633-3874, Fax: 212-633-3820, e-mail: reprints@elsevier.com.

The *Surgical Clinics of North America* is also published in Spanish by McGraw-Hill Interamericana Editores S.A., P.O. Box 5-237 06500 Mexico D.F. Mexico; and in Portuguese by Interlivros Edicoes Ltda., Rua Comandante Coelho 1085, CEP 21250, Rio de Janeiro, Brazil; and in Greek by Paschalidis Medical Publications, Athens Greece.

The *Surgical Clinics of North America* is covered in *MEDLINE/PubMed (Index Medicus), EMBASE/Excerpta Medica, Current Contents/Clinical Medicine, Current Contents/Life Sciences, Science Citation Index,* and *ISI/BIOMED.*

Printed and bound by CPI Group (UK) Ltd, Croydon, CR0 4YY

Transferred to digital print 2012

Contributors

CONSULTING EDITOR

RONALD F. MARTIN, MD, FACS
Staff Surgeon, Department of Surgery, Marshfield Clinic, Marshfield; Clinical Associate
Professor, University of Wisconsin School of Medicine and Public Health, Madison,
Wisconsin; Colonel, Medical Corps, United States Army Reserve

EDITOR

A. OSAMA GABER, MD, FACS
J.C. Walter Jr. Distinguished Endowed Chair, Director, Methodist J.C. Walter Jr.
Transplant Center; Vice Chair, Department of Surgery, Houston Methodist Hospital,
Houston, Texas; Professor of Surgery, Weill Cornell Medical College, New York, New York

AUTHORS

RITA R. ALLOWAY, PharmD, FCCP
Research Professor of Medicine, Division of Nephrology, Department of Internal Medicine,
University of Cincinnati College of Medicine, Cincinnati, Ohio

EMAD H. ASHAM, MD, FRCS
Abdominal Transplant & Hepatopancreatobiliary Surgeon, Department of Surgery,
Methodist J.C. Walter Jr. Transplant Center, Houston Methodist Hospital, Texas Medical
Center, Houston, Texas

MEREDITH J. AULL, PharmD
Assistant Research Professor of Pharmacology in Surgery, Division of Transplant Surgery,
NewYork-Presbyterian/Weill Cornell Medical Center, New York, New York

LOKESH BATHLA, MD
Fellow, Section of Transplant Surgery, University of Nebraska Medical Center, Omaha,
Nebraska

LORENA BEJARANO-PINEDA, MD
Division of Transplantation, Department of Surgery, University of Illinois at Chicago,
Chicago, Illinois

ENRICO BENEDETTI, MD
Division of Transplantation, Department of Surgery, University of Illinois at Chicago,
Chicago, Illinois

DAVID P. BERNARD, MBA/MHA, FACHE
Methodist J.C. Walter Jr. Transplant Center; Vice President, Houston Methodist Hospital,
Houston, Texas

FRANCESCO BIANCO, MD
Division of Minimally Invasive and Robotic Surgery, Department of Surgery, University of
Illinois at Chicago, Chicago, Illinois

BRIAN A. BRUCKNER, MD
Department of Cardiovascular Surgery, Methodist DeBakey Heart & Vascular Center, Houston Methodist Hospital, Houston, Texas

WIDA CHERIKH, PhD
United Network for Organ Sharing, Richmond, Virginia

MARCELO CYPEL, MD, MSc
Toronto Lung Transplant Program, Toronto General Hospital, University Health Network, University of Toronto, Toronto, Ontario, Canada

RICHARD N. FORMICA, MD
Departments of Internal Medicine and Surgery, Yale University School of Medicine, New Haven, Connecticut

JOHN J. FRIEDEWALD, MD
Comprehensive Transplant Center, Department of Surgery, Feinberg School of Medicine, Northwestern University, Chicago, Illinois

LILLIAN W. GABER, MD
Department of Pathology and Genomic Medicine, Houston Methodist Hospital, Houston, Texas; Professor, Department of Pathology, Weill Cornell Medical College, New York, New York

A. OSAMA GABER, MD, FACS
J.C. Walter Jr. Distinguished Endowed Chair, Director, Methodist J.C. Walter Jr. Transplant Center; Vice Chair, Department of Surgery, Houston Methodist Hospital, Houston, Texas; Professor of Surgery, Weill Cornell Medical College, New York, New York

RAQUEL GARCIA-ROCA, MD
Division of Transplantation, Department of Surgery, University of Illinois at Chicago, Chicago, Illinois

R. MARK GHOBRIAL, MD, PhD, FACS, FRCS
Director, Center for Liver Disease & Professor of Surgery, Department of Surgery, Methodist J.C. Walter Jr. Transplant Center, Houston Methodist Hospital, Texas Medical Center, Houston, Texas

PIER C. GIULIANOTTI, MD
Division of Minimally Invasive and Robotic Surgery, Department of Surgery, University of Illinois at Chicago, Chicago, Illinois

AJAY K. ISRANI, MD, MS
Scientific Registry of Transplant Recipients, Minneapolis Medical Research Foundation; Division of Nephrology, Department of Medicine, Hennepin County Medical Center; Department of Epidemiology and Community Health, School of Public Health, University of Minnesota, Minneapolis, Minnesota

HOONBAE JEON, MD
Division of Transplantation, Department of Surgery, University of Illinois at Chicago, Chicago, Illinois

SANDIP KAPUR, MD, FACS
Associate Professor of Surgery, G. Tom Shires, M.D. Faculty Scholar in Surgery, Chief, Division of Transplant Surgery, New York-Presbyterian/Weill Cornell Medical Center, New York, New York

AHMED KASEB, MD
Assistant Professor of Medicine, Department of Gastrointestinal Medical Oncology, The University of Texas MD Anderson Cancer Center, Houston, Texas

BERTRAM L. KASISKE, MD
Scientific Registry of Transplant Recipients, Minneapolis Medical Research Foundation; Division of Nephrology, Department of Medicine, Hennepin County Medical Center, Minneapolis, Minnesota

SHAF KESHAVJEE, MD, MSc
Toronto Lung Transplant Program, Toronto General Hospital, University Health Network, University of Toronto, Toronto, Ontario, Canada

RICHARD J. KNIGHT, MD
Department of Surgery, Houston Methodist Hospital, Houston, Texas; Professor, Department of Surgery, Weill Cornell Medical College, New York, New York

ALAN LANGNAS, DO
Professor, Chief of Transplant Surgery, University of Nebraska Medical Center, Omaha, Nebraska

MATTHIAS LOEBE, MD, PhD
Department of Cardiovascular Surgery, Methodist DeBakey Heart & Vascular Center, Houston Methodist Hospital, Houston, Texas

TIAGO N. MACHUCA, MD, PhD
Toronto Lung Transplant Program, Toronto General Hospital, University Health Network, University of Toronto, Toronto, Ontario, Canada

LINDA W. MOORE, MS, RD, CCRP
Director, Research Programs, Department of Surgery, Houston Methodist Hospital Physician Organization, Houston, Texas

JOSÉ OBERHOLZER, MD
Division of Transplantation, Department of Surgery, University of Illinois at Chicago, Chicago, Illinois

SAMIR J. PATEL, PharmD
Department of Pharmacy, Houston Methodist Hospital, Houston, Texas

LIMAEL E. RODRIGUEZ, MD
Department of Cardiovascular Surgery, Methodist DeBakey Heart & Vascular Center, Houston Methodist Hospital, Houston, Texas

BASMA SADAKA, PharmD, MsCR, BCPS
Division of Nephrology, Department of Internal Medicine, University of Cincinnati College of Medicine, Cincinnati, Ohio

CIARA J. SAMANA, MSPH
United Network for Organ Sharing, Richmond, Virginia

ROBERTA L. SCHWARTZ, MHS
Executive Vice President, Houston Methodist Hospital, Houston, Texas

VADIM SHERMAN, MD, FRCSC, FACS
Medical Director, Bariatric and Metabolic Surgery Center, Department of Surgery, Houston Methodist Hospital, Houston, Texas; Assistant Professor, Department of Surgery, Weill Cornell Medical College, New York, New York

DARREN STEWART, MS
United Network for Organ Sharing, Richmond, Virginia

ERIK E. SUAREZ, MD
Department of Cardiovascular Surgery, Methodist DeBakey Heart & Vascular Center, Houston Methodist Hospital, Houston, Texas

NABIL TARIQ, MD, FACS
Bariatric and Metabolic Surgery Center, Department of Surgery, Houston Methodist Hospital, Houston, Texas; Assistant Professor, Department of Surgery, Weill Cornell Medical College, New York, New York

IVO TZVETANOV, MD
Assistant Professor of Surgery, Division of Transplantation, Department of Surgery, University of Illinois at Chicago, Chicago, Illinois

LUCIANO M. VARGAS, MD
Assistant Professor of Surgery, Section of Transplant Surgery, University of Nebraska Medical Center, Omaha, Nebraska

E. STEVE WOODLE, MD, FACS
Division of Transplantation, Department of Surgery, University of Cincinnati College of Medicine, Cincinnati, Ohio

SUSAN ZYLICZ, RN, BSN, MBA
Director, Methodist J.C. Walter Jr. Transplant Center, Houston Methodist Hospital, Houston, Texas

Contents

The response to allografting involves adaptive and innate immune mechanisms. In the adaptive system, activated T cells differentiate to cytotoxic
effectors that attack the graft and trigger B cells to differentiation to plasma
cells that produce anti-HLA antibodies. The innate immune system recognizes antigens in a non-specific manner and recruits immune cells to the
graft through the productions of chemotactic factors, and activation of
cytokines and the complement cascade. In the kidney the tubules and
the endothelium are the targets of the rejection response. Immune suppression is effective in modulating the adaptive immune system effect
on graft histology.

Robotic-assisted surgery has enabled organ transplantation in a minimally
invasive fashion. Kidney transplantation is the best treatment of patients
with chronic renal failure. Robotic surgery has reduced the difficulties
associated with kidney transplantation for obese patients. Benefits such
as reduced recovery period and reduced number of wound complications
and surgical site infections have been attained with the robotic surgical
approach. We believe that robotic-assisted surgery has expanded the
ability to complete complex surgical procedures in a minimally invasive
fashion. However, advanced training and experience are required in all
surgeons who are interested in pursuing this technique.

Despite its vast potential, concerns about donor safety continue to limit the
expansion of living-donor liver transplantation (LDLT) in Western countries.
In light of the technical refinements, relatively lower risk of complications
with left lobe (LL) LDLT with comparable outcomes, and the overriding
concern for donor safety, there is renewed interest in using LL allograft
as the first choice for LDLT; thereby, fundamentally shifting the risks of
LDLT from the donor to the recipient. There is ample evidence that LL
LDLT when performed with graft inflow modification where indicated,
has long-term outcomes as good as cadaveric LT.

> Much of the success of left ventricular assist devices (LVAD) can be attributed to the second-generation HeartMate II (Thoratec, Pleasanton, CA, USA), which is the most commonly used device to date. The latest generation of LVADs is currently undergoing clinical trials worldwide. Developers have focused on improving the limitations of the second generation with emphasis on enhancing efficiency further, decreasing complications, and increasing ease of implantability. Clinical management of a patient with an LVAD is also an excellent example of the multidisciplinary approach of care that is undoubtedly the future of medicine.

> Morbid obesity increases the risk of complications and allograft failure in transplant patients. Bariatric surgery is both safe and effective in patients with chronic kidney disease and end-stage renal disease, improves eligibility for transplant based on body mass index, and does not affect postoperative immunosuppressant dosing regimens. Bariatric surgery in patients with liver disease has been shown to be safe and effective, although they remain at high risk in the setting of portal hypertension. Sleeve gastrectomy may become increasingly used both pretransplant and posttransplant, as it can result in low complication rates and excellent weight loss, and retains intestinal continuity.

> After a brief review of conventional lung preservation, this article discusses the rationale behind ex vivo lung perfusion and how it has shifted the paradigm of organ preservation from conventional static cold ischemia to the utilization of functional normothermia, restoring the lung's own metabolism and its reparative processes. Technical aspects and previous clinical experience as well as opportunities to address specific donor organ injuries in a personalized medicine approach are also reviewed.

> The current kidney allocation system for transplants is outdated and has not evolved to reflect the changing demographics of patients on the waiting list. This article proposes a new system for kidney allocation, which more appropriately incorporates the biology of highly sensitized patients into the waiting-time scoring algorithm. This system will significantly reduce mismatches between possible donor kidney longevity and life expectancy of recipients, and makes incremental advances toward more geographic sharing. The proposed system makes significant progress toward eliminating deficiencies in the current system, and has the potential to increase the supply of available kidneys.

Current Topics in Transplantation

SURGICAL CLINICS
OF NORTH AMERICA

ISSUE OF RELATED INTEREST

Clinics in Chest Medicine June 2011 (Vol. 32, Issue 2)
Lung Transplantation
Robert M. Kotloff, MD, *Editor*

**DOWNLOAD
Free App!**

Review Articles
THE CLINICS

NOW AVAILABLE FOR YOUR iPhone and iPad

Foreword
Current Topics in Transplantation

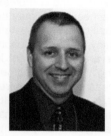

Ronald F. Martin, MD, FACS
Consulting Editor

There comes a time in many surgeons' careers where the demands of running the business of patient care becomes more challenging than the actual caring for the patients. I suspect it is inevitable that we should all develop in such a way that performing our daily tasks of diagnosing and treating the sick becomes easier and perhaps even comfortable. After all, although our understanding of how humans medically function or fail to—and what we can do to prevent or alter that—evolves apace, the rate of change of medical knowledge pales in comparison to the pace of change for the society in which we provide the care. One stroke of a pen or even the threat of a penstroke in Washington, DC can set our entire workplace on its ear.

For the past several years, I have had the privilege of being part of a small group of doctors who are responsible for running our fairly good-sized organization. During that time we had the market collapse of 2008, the persistent effect of two lingering armed conflicts in Asia, a significant decline in the manufacturing economy (which greatly affected our local patient population), somewhat polarized transitions of both state and federal executive administrations and legislative branches, and a host of other "nonmedical" frame shifts with which to contend. However, none of those features has seemed all that onerous to work around or with from my standpoint. Change is always the nature of the game. What I do find particularly challenging is one somewhat related concept: the shift from volume-based care to value-based care and how to get doctors to buy into it.

At its core, value-based care and volume-based care should not even be a transition—should it? If we were always doing thing *for* patients as opposed to doing things *to* patients, we would *always* be providing value-based care. We would always be considering the health risk and benefit consequences of all clinical decisions in the context of the affordability and effectiveness of the care for the patient. And if we really thought and acted this way—in an ideal world—value-based care would be all that we would deliver. But we don't practice that way. Intentionally or unintentionally, we

Surg Clin N Am 93 (2013) xi–xiii
http://dx.doi.org/10.1016/j.suc.2013.09.005
0039-6109/13/$ – see front matter © 2013 Published by Elsevier Inc.

provide incentives for behavior, and overwhelmingly, but not surprisingly, that is the behavior we are most likely to see.

For the most part, doctors and other organizations are reimbursed for what they do. More accurately, we are generally reimbursed for what we meant to do or claimed to do. Although many schemes to bundle, risk-share, and cost-share exist in many forms, pay for play is still the rule. Indication, efficacy, and quality are to some degree implicitly accepted. Or at least they were. At varying degrees of speed and completeness, measures of quality are entering into reimbursement schemes. There may be some who claim we try to evaluate indication but I have never really seen any system that tries that can't be gamed to the point of uselessness. Efficacy is also an illusory target for two main reasons: we probably don't know what we are talking about in the first place and even if we did we aren't that good at measuring it. Some outcomes are pretty reliable (eg, survival). After that, the reliability of the measure and measurement degrades rapidly. It is hard to say who is truly disease free, for example. Quality of life gets a lot of chatter but that gets pretty subjective as well. Not to mention that some parameters that we (institutionalized medicine) claim as goals for patients (cessation of smoking, weight reduction, alcohol consumption) are not necessarily in line with what some patients want. So in that case, who is right? Is it the consumer or the provider of the service or care? Is it the recipient of the care or the recipient of the bill? Furthermore, who gets to decide: the individual, the family, the provider, the insurer, the co-insured, state government, federal government, or other?

Our current buzzword is "accountable care." Accountable to whom and for what, I am not quite sure. It appears to me that the purpose of accountable care is to achieve one major goal that has little to do with accountability or care: "accountable care" or its mechanistic constructs, accountable care organizations, make it possible for a commercial or government payer to pay less global money for a service without having to admit to any specific entity that they are being discounted. In effect, the payer can simply claim that any individual entity can make as much as it ever did, maybe more. The entity just has to climb in the gladiatorial ring with the other partners and take the lost money from them. Simple. The payer doesn't pick winners or losers, it's just Darwinism. The payer keeps a little more for its needs and the providers can scrap over the rest.

Dear reader, please don't misunderstand me; I don't actually have a problem with the government or commercial payers doing this to us. Well, maybe a little problem with the commercial payers. We in medicine have known for decades that we had an unsustainable model, yet we frustrated every other attempt to change it to the best of our ability. One might say that the reckoning has come but that would be optimistic. These current changes are too poorly informed and ill equipped or designed to address the real systemic issues. Most likely this will be another step along the path to something more effective. What I do take issue with in these current large political shifts is that they are based far more on hopes, beliefs, and ideologies than they are on facts. And facts are stubborn things.

To borrow from Lord Kelvin, "To measure is to know." I suggest that we have to go further than that. We need not only to measure but we need to measure, analyze, and share. There are many barriers to that. The usual barriers of protected health information are usually surmountable with de-identification tools. The more difficult barriers are the ones in which the data can be used to alter business relationships, especially when payers and providers are using the same data pipelines. I think we can safely say there are some significant trust issues in our business.

Our friends in the transplant world have long been the leaders in many things. They excel at patient care and in my view are unparalleled in their commitment to patients and team. Perhaps more important is that our transplant community shares information better than any of the rest of us. Even though no system is perfect, the transplant community is as transparent as any portion of medical care. We all have much to learn from them in terms of patient care and systems control.

Dr Gaber and his colleagues have compiled an extraordinary collection of reviews. The expertise reflected in these articles comes at the expense of tireless work and commitment. We are deeply indebted to them for sharing this experience with us and for their example of what can be done when we truly work as an organization that holds ourselves accountable.

Ronald F. Martin, MD, FACS
Department of Surgery
Marshfield Clinic
1000 North Oak Avenue
Marshfield, WI 54449, USA

E-mail address:
martin.ronald@marshfieldclinic.org

Preface

Current Topics in Transplantation

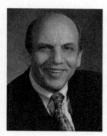

A. Osama Gaber, MD, FACS
Editor

The evolution of transplantation as a discipline represents one of the earliest and most successful examples of translational science. Surgical pioneers such as Joseph Murray and David Hume applied the immunologic discoveries made in the laboratories of Sir Peter Medawar and his colleagues to create the first series of human kidney transplants. The surgical field that was birthed out of the work of these and other pioneering surgeons has prospered into modern transplantation and led to saving hundreds of thousands of lives, and to the advancement of surgical sciences and human health.

The early surgical pioneers were also keenly aware of the multidisciplinary nature of the emerging surgical discipline and presented to surgery some of the earliest examples of the success of such an endeavor. This awareness was best described by Thomas Starzl in the inaugural presidential address of the American Society of Transplant Surgeons in 1974, when he stated that "so far the field of clinical transplantation has grown up in what might be termed a giant multidisciplinary matrix." In the same address Starzl spoke about what he then considered the obvious danger to transplantation, "so has been at least one possible disadvantage, which is the potential disconnection of our specialty from a traditional base." And he continued, "The arrangement to publish our proceedings in a surgical journal will remind of our origins in surgery." This danger of dislodging transplantation away from its surgical roots remains a concern even today and it is with this background in mind that the current issue of the *Surgical Clinics of North America* has been approached. Our general goal was to respond to the call made from the stage of the first meeting of transplant surgeons and to present the latest advances in the transplantation field to the general community of surgeons.

The articles selected for this issue highlight the unique scientific underpinnings of transplantation, its surgical complexity, multidisciplinary scope, complex regulatory and business environment, and also its future potential and challenges. L. Gaber and her colleagues, for example, discuss the emerging role of the innate immune

Surg Clin N Am 93 (2013) xv–xvi
http://dx.doi.org/10.1016/j.suc.2013.09.004
0039-6109/13/$ – see front matter © 2013 Elsevier Inc. All rights reserved.

system in transplant early function and transplant rejection, a topic of great interest to all surgeons, particularly considering the potential role of the innate immune system and its activation in ischemia-reperfusion injury and in sepsis-mediated injury. Further enriching our understanding of the immune response, Dr Basma and the Cincinnati group describe the B-Cell and antibody mediated mechanism of transplant rejection. We also discuss the emerging role of bariatric surgery in the preparation of organ failure patients for transplantation, the complex distribution systems for deceased organ transplants, and the new networks being formed to facilitate donor exchanges. With the expanded use of left ventricular assist devices, we outline the potential general surgical complications and emergencies in these patients. We outline advances in the management of patients with hepatocellular carcinoma and hopefully enrich the surgical debate about the management of these complex patients. Dr Keshavjee and his group describe their progress towards lung preservation. Finally, we are privileged to be able to include an article by the group from the University of Illinois describing the use of robotic techniques to perform kidney transplantation, and another from the University of Nebraska describing the procedure of adult-to-adult left lobe transplants. In every article we have emphasized relevance to the practicing surgeon and to the surgical resident so each may grasp the principles of care of this unique population.

Presenting this issue to the general surgery community gives me and the other contributors special pleasure as we all remember fondly the special place the *Surgical Clinics of North America* had in our own education. Making an issue like this possible is a testament to the dedication of the staff of the *Surgical Clinics of North America*, and the series editor, John Vassallo. The authors would like to thank them all for their emphasis on delivering the highest quality issue and their continued support throughout the production process.

Finally, I would like to quote from the presidential address given by Anthony Monaco, the 12th president of the American Society of Transplant Surgeons: "Transplantation is a vibrant, vital field, ever changing, ever challenging, ever stimulating, ever accomplishing, with many limitless possibilities to affect all aspects of medicine and surgery." In this statement, Dr Monaco encapsulates the spirit of modern transplantation and explains why transplant surgeons continue to advocate passionately for their discipline and their patients.

A. Osama Gaber, MD, FACS
Department of Surgery
Houston Methodist Hospital
6550 Fannin Street, Suite 1661
Houston, TX 77030, USA

E-mail address:
aogaber@houstonmethodist.org

Personal note from the editor: I would like to give special thanks to two chairs of surgery that understood transplantation and its contribution to the field of surgery, and supported keeping it part of the surgical discipline: Barbara L. Bass and Louis G. Britt.

A Surgeons' Guide to Renal Transplant Immunopathology, Immunology, and Immunosuppression

Lillian W. Gaber, MD[a],*, Richard J. Knight, MD[b],
Samir J. Patel, PharmD[c]

KEYWORDS

- Immune suppression • Graft rejection • Biopsy • Adaptive immune responses

KEY POINTS

- The response to allografting involves both the adaptive and innate immune systems. In the adaptive immune system, T cells become activated upon recognition of alloantigens presented by donor and host antigen-presenting cells (APCs).
- Activated T cells can help B-cell differentiation to antibody producing plasma cells and memory cells. Antibody mediated rejection is triggered when enough circulating antibodies to allograft antigens are present or are produced.
- The innate immune system recognizes antigens and pathogens in a non-specific manner and its functions include removal of foreign substances and recruiting immune cells through the productions of chemotactic factors, and activation of cytokines and the complement cascade.
- In the kidney, Immune activation leads to targeting of the tubules and the endothelium by allo-stimulated cells. Based on the timing of its occurrence rejection was classified as hyperacute, accelerated acute, acute and chronic. These terminologies have been replaced by the Banff group with a more histological nomenclature.
- Immune suppressive medications are introduced during the induction phase and closely monitored in the adjustment phase to prevent early rejection. Following that the chronic maintenance phase of immune suppression is characterized by step wise decrease in medication doses and possibly by withdrawal of one or more of them.

[a] Department of Pathology and Genomic Medicine, Houston Methodist Hospital, 6565 Fannin Street, Houston, TX 77030, USA; [b] Department of Surgery, Houston Methodist Hospital, 6550 Fannin Street, Houston, TX 77030, USA; [c] Department of Pharmacy, Houston Methodist Hospital, 6565 Fannin Street, Houston, TX 77030, USA
* Corresponding author.
E-mail address: lgaber@houstonmethodist.org

Surg Clin N Am 93 (2013) 1293–1307
http://dx.doi.org/10.1016/j.suc.2013.09.002
0039-6109/13/$ – see front matter © 2013 Elsevier Inc. All rights reserved.

surgical.theclinics.com

The immune system response to allografting is a multistep process that involves both the adaptive and innate immune systems. In the adaptive immune system, T cells become activated on recognition of alloantigens presented by donor and host antigen-presenting cells (APCs).[1] T-cell activation results in the activation and recruitment of other cell types, and in T-Cell maturation to effector cells, which induce tissue destruction and the production of cytokines.[2]

The innate immune system comprises cells that recognize and respond to antigens and pathogens in a nonspecific manner, and without conferring long-lasting protective immunity. The major functions of the innate immune system include recruiting immune cells through the production of chemotactic factors and cytokines, activation of the complement cascade, identification and removal of foreign substances, and acting as a physical and chemical barrier to foreign agents. One of the most important functions of the innate immune system is the activation of the adaptive immune system through a process known as antigen presentation. In the allograft, ischemia reperfusion–induced oxidative allograft injury can lead to generation of damage-associated molecules, such as heat shock protein 72, high mobility group box 1, and a hyaluronan fragment. All of these molecules act as endogenous ligands of toll-like receptors and are recognized by intragraft toll-like receptor 4–bearing and toll-like receptor 2–bearing dendritic cells. Stimulated dendritic cells mature and initiate cytokine-driven development of the recipient's adaptive alloimmune response. This same mechanism has been implicated in the development of accelerated atherosclerosis of the allograft and chronic rejection via injury-induced proliferation of smooth muscle cells.[3,4] Recent evidence has shown that brain death is a powerful trigger of cytokine storms. Besides inducing organ damage, cytokines recruit inflammatory cells into organs that accentuate the damage and are instrumental in mediating the manifestations of ischemic damage. Allograft injury, induced by the reperfusion response, initiates an innate immune response by activating innate immune cells (such as donor-derived and recipient-derived toll-like receptor–bearing dendritic cells and innate lymphocytes natural killer cells, dendritic cells, and macrophages) as well as humoral factors (complement, natural IgM antibodies).[5] These innate immune cells act as inflammatory cells promoting rejection by directly damaging the graft. Alternatively, the acute innate intragraft inflammatory response can initiate and expand the adaptive alloimmune system, because the innate inflammatory cells act as APCs to the different major histocompatibility complex (MHC) antigens. Innate immune cells can also regulate differentiation of T effector cells by the virtue of their cytokine production, thus affecting the nature and strength of the rejection response.[6] The impact of innate immune system activation on tolerance development is also 2 sided, because some cell types promote tolerance induction by eliminating donor APCs.[7] The cytokine milieu created by the activation of innate immune cells can be detrimental to the induction of Foxp3+ regulatory T cells, a key cell type involved in transplant tolerance.[8]

Most of the immune targets in an allograft are the polymorphic HLA molecules. Class I HLA antigens are expressed in all nucleated cells, such as tubular cells, and interact with CD8+ T cells. HLA class II molecules are expressed on activated cells and on APCs. T cells are activated by graft antigens either directly through crosslinking with HLA molecules or more commonly indirectly via interacting with APCs that are processing donor antigen. This interaction requires engagement of the cell receptor and accessory activation molecules. T-cell activation results in expression of T-cell activation markers, secretion of cytokines such as interleukin 2 (IL-2), leading to activation and mobilization of CD4+ and CD8+ cells into the graft, and creates the conditions prompting graft infiltration.[9]

Activated T cells can also help B cells, which in response to antigenic stimulation are triggered into differentiation to antibody-producing plasma cells and memory cells. Conversely, there is some evidence that T-cell depletion early after transplantation in patients receiving some of the depleting antibodies may cause increased levels of the B-cell cytokine BAFF.[10] Calcineurin inhibitors (CNIs) may also hold B cells in a transitional state, and weaning of CNIs may release B cells to become fully activated and differentiate.[11] Once B cells are activated, memory cells maintain the sensitization memory for the inciting HLA antigen, and plasma cell activation produces anti-HLA antibodies. Antibody-mediated rejection (ABMR) is triggered when enough circulating antibodies to allograft antigens are present or are produced. Antigen-antibody interaction and their deposition in the graft lead to complement activation and triggering of an inflammatory response centered on endothelial surfaces of the peritubular and glomerular capillaries.[12]

In addition, T-cell activation induces activation of cytokines and other inflammatory mediators, both within the interstitium and around blood vessels. This activation results in upregulation of vascular endothelial adhesion molecules, which attract inflammatory cells into the vascular space. Graft infiltrating cells recognize class I alloantigens on donor tubular cells, whereas vascular endothelial cells express both class I and class II MHC antigens. Inflammatory activation of the endothelium increases the intensity of class II expression and may also accentuate the expression of other alloantigens, such as endothelial-monocyte antigens, and other polymorphic alloantigen systems, which can be particularly important in the evolution of vascular rejection.[13]

CLINICAL MANIFESTATIONS OF TRANSPLANT REJECTION

The result of immune system activation is the targeting of the allograft tissue by allostimulated cells. In the kidney, the tubules, the endothelium, or both are the main targets for the inflammatory antigen-specific immune response. This immune injury is manifested clinically by reduction in excretory capacity of the kidney with decreased urine output and increase in serum creatinine level. Endothelial swelling and injury result in reduction in blood flow and development of manifestation of tubular necrosis. On examination, there is kidney swelling, tenderness, and possibly fever, proteinuria, and hematuria.[14] These classic clinical manifestations of rejection have almost disappeared with the newer immune suppressants, leaving frequent monitoring of function and repeated biopsies as the only effective means to monitor for rejection besides changes in serum creatinine level.[15]

REJECTION CLASSIFICATION

Based on the timing of its occurrence, rejection was classified as hyperacute, accelerated acute, acute, and chronic. Although these terminologies have been replaced by more histologic nomenclature, they still provide a useful guide to the cause and progression of rejection. Hyperacute rejection started immediately after perfusion and was related to the presence of high levels of antidonor antibodies, the deposition of which on the vascular endothelium led to complement activation and intravascular thrombosis. Advances in antibody detection by single antigen beads have almost eliminated this type of rejection.[16] Accelerated acute rejection was usually diagnosed in patients with preexisting antibodies in whom antibody levels had decreased over time. Usually, the graft works for a few days, then an anamnestic immune response is mounted by the sensitized host. Immune activation leads to florid production of antibodies and endothelial cell injury. Acute rejection described the rejection occurring usually early after the transplant and characterized by the lymphocytic infiltration whether in the tubules (acute cellular rejection) or the blood vessels (acute vascular rejection [AVR]). Chronic rejection was believed to be related to chronic slow antibody deposition, leading to progressive vascular sclerosis of the allograft.

DESIGN OF IMMUNE SUPPRESSION PROTOCOLS

Because all immune suppressants possess significant side effects, immunosuppression protocols are based on the simultaneous use of multiple drugs. This strategy achieves immune suppression efficacy without having to use any of the drugs in full, toxic doses. After transplantation, the induction phase of immunosuppression is achieved by administration of biological agents. Immune-suppressive medications are introduced during the induction phase and closely monitored in the adjustment phase to prevent early rejection. After that, the chronic maintenance phase of immune suppression is characterized by stepwise decrease in medication doses and possibly by withdrawal of 1 or more of them.

BIOLOGICAL AGENTS

Biological agents include both monoclonal and polyclonal antibodies. A monoclonal antibody is derived from a single cell line that is reactive with a single epitope. The most commonly used monoclonal antibody in clinical transplantation is basiliximab, a chimeric mouse-human monoclonal antibody to the α chain (CD25) of the IL-2 receptor of T cells. A polyclonal antibody is made up of a combination of immunoglobulin molecules that identify different epitopes on the same cells or different antigenic determinants on multiple cells. Thymoglobulin, a rabbit antithymocyte globulin, is the most widely used polyclonal antibody. Thymoglobulin and some monoclonal antibodies such as alemtuzamab remove lymphocytes from the peripheral circulation and are thus classified as depleting antibodies. The cells may be removed by several different mechanisms, including complement-mediated lysis or reticuloendothelial-dependent phagocytosis. The effects of depleting antibodies tend to be long lasting. In the case of thymoglobulin and alemtuzamab, it takes several months for the peripheral T-cell count to return to normal after treatment.[17] Conversely, nondepleting antibodies inactivate the target cell but do not remove it from the circulation. An example of a nondepleting antibody is basiliximab. By binding to the IL-2 receptor, it effectively inhibits the cell from responding to IL-2, but the T cell remains in the peripheral circulation.

These 3 biological agents (basiliximab, alemtuzamab, and thymoglobulin) are all used in induction of immune suppression. Thymoglobulin is also used for the treatment of acute rejection. The success of thymoglobulin has been attributed to the large number of antibodies and targets that it recognizes, including immune response antigens, adhesion and cell trafficking epitopes, and multiple heterogeneous pathway antigens. Thymoglobulin is the preferred induction agent in recipients at high immunologic risk and in patients with delayed graft function, in whom the introduction of nephrotoxic immunosuppressants has to be delayed until kidney function recovers.[18] Alemtuzamab is a humanized depleting antibody that targets both T and B cells by binding to the CD-52 receptor on the surface of lymphocytes. Alemtuzamab is used also as an induction agent, generally in patients with a similar profile to those requiring thymoglobulin.[19]

Rituximab is another depleting humanized antibody that binds to the CD-20 receptor on B cells. It is used for desensitization of recipients with preformed HLA antibodies before transplantation, as part of multimodality treatment of antibody-mediated acute rejection, and as a therapy for recurrent glomerular disease after transplantation. Recently, there have been trials to use rituximab in induction of sensitized patients, and the results seem encouraging.[20]

Another newly introduced biological agent, eculizumab, is a humanized monoclonal antibody that is unique among biological agents used in transplantation. Eculizumab does not bind to lymphocytes but acts on the complement system through binding to complement component C5, resulting in effective inhibition of the complement cascade. Based on its mechanism of action, it has predictably been considered a potential adjunctive agent for the prevention or treatment of antibody-mediated acute rejection. A recent preliminary study of its use in induction therapy for patients with flow crossmatch-positive kidney transplants has stimulated the conduct of a phase 3 randomized trial for that same indication.[12]

MAINTENANCE IMMUNOSUPPRESSION

Maintenance immunosuppressive agents have traditionally been pharmacologic agents used for long-term immunosuppression. Pharmacologic immunosuppression is divided into 4 groups: corticosteroids, CNIs (such as cyclosporine and tacrolimus), mammalian target of rapamycin (mTOR) inhibitors (including sirolimus and everolimus), and the antimetabolites (including mycophenolate mofetil and azathioprine). These drugs are used to prevent T-cell–mediated acute rejection. A useful way to understand their function is to consider these agents as lymphocyte cell cycle inhibitors.

THE LYMPHOCYTE CELL CYCLE

G0 is the resting stage of the cell. T lymphocytes exist for most of their life span in this state. In order to proliferate, cells must reenter the G1 phase, in which a variety of proteins, including cytokines, are synthesized in preparation for DNA synthesis.[21] In the S phase, DNA synthesis and replication result in each chromosome producing 2 identical chromatids. A second gap or G2 phase allows the final cytoplasmic reorganizations required for cellular division to occur. The M (mitotic) phase then involves chromosomal condensation, breakdown of the nuclear membrane, separation of the sister chromatids, generation of 2 new nuclei, and division of the cytoplasm to form 2 daughter cells. A typical lymphocyte cell cycle may take 12 to 16 hours to complete, with several additional hours initially required to take the cell from G0 to G1.[22,23]

CALCINEURIN INHIBITORS (CNIs)

The CNIs are cyclosporine and tacrolimus, which, although structurally distinct, act to block the synthesis of proinflammatory cytokines through the inhibition of calcineurin. The activity of tacrolimus in vitro is 10 to 100 times greater than that of cyclosporine. Both cyclosporine A (CsA) and tacrolimus are prodrugs; in order to gain pharmacologic activity they must bind to cytoplasmic components termed immunophilins. The immunophilins are cytoplasmic enzymes; cyclophilin, which binds to CsA, and FK-binding protein 12 (FKBP12), which binds to tacrolimus.

T-CELL SIGNALING AND CALCINEURIN INHIBITION

The T-cell receptor recognizes foreign antigen in combination with an APC. This recognition event is transferred from the cell membrane to the cell interior via the CD3 membrane complex. This signal initiates a programmed series of phosphorylations of membrane-associated and cytoplasmic kinases. These events cause a rapid and sustained increase in cytosolic calcium via influx through surface channels and release from intracellular membrane stores. Increases in intracellular calcium concentration stimulate the catalytic activity of the phosphatase calcineurin. The best-defined target of calcineurin activity is the nuclear factor of activated T cells (NF-AT). Calcineurin causes dephosphorylation of NF-AT and carries the product through the nuclear membrane. Once in the nucleus, NF-AT serves as the primary regulatory protein that promotes the transcription of IL-2 (**Fig. 1**).[24]

Thus, the CsA-cyclophilin and the tacrolimus-FK binding complexes block T-cell activation by binding to the phosphatase calcineurin, forming an inhibitory association, which thereby dampens the dephosphorylation, transport, and release of NF-AT in the nucleus. As a consequence of these events, entry in to the cell cycle is arrested at the G0 or G1 phase, synthesis of DNA, RNA, is inhibited, and cytokine production is abrogated. This is not the only mechanism of action of the CNIs. Both CsA and tacrolimus also enhance the expression of transforming growth factor β, a cytokine that has not only immunosuppressive effects but causes renal allograft fibrosis.

mTOR INHIBITORS

Like the CNIs, sirolimus is a prodrug and binds to the same protein as tacrolimus, FKBP12, but at a different site. The enzyme target of this complex is mTOR, a 289-kDa serine-threonine kinase. Whereas the calcineurin inhibitors act early at the G0 to G1 phase to block IL-2 transcription, sirolimus acts later at the G1 stage of the cell cycle to block the T-cell response to IL-2, resulting in inhibition of protein synthesis.

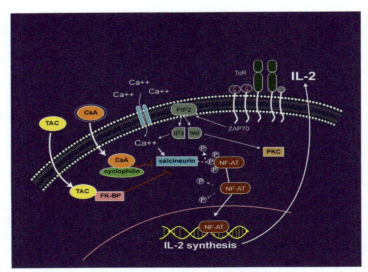

Fig. 1. Cyclosporine (CsA) and tacrolimus (TAC) are prodrugs that bind to cytoplasmic immunophilins: cyclophilin binds to CsA, and FKBP12 (FK binding protein) binds to tacrolimus. The drug-immunophilin complexes block the phosphatase activity of calcineurin; the best-defined target of calcineurin activity is Nuclear factor of activated T cells (NF-AT). Calcineurin causes dephosphorylation of NF-AT, affecting the transcription of interleukin -2(IL-2). Thus, the calcineurin inhibitors interfere with T-cell cycle progression from G0 to G1. DAG, diacylglycerol; IP3, Inositol trisphosphate; PIP2, Phosphatidylinositol 4,5-bisphosphate; PKC, protein kinase C; TcR, T-cell receptor; ZAP 70, Zeta-chain-associated protein kinase 70.

T-CELL SIGNALING AND mTOR INHIBITION

First, IL-2 binding to the IL-2 receptor (CD25) on T cells results in activation of phosphoinositide-3-OH kinase to generate phosphatidylinositol 3,4,5 triphosphate. This molecule, in turn, activates the serine-threonine protein kinase Akt. Once activated, Akt relieves the inhibitory effect of the tuberous sclerosis complex proteins TSC1 and TSC2 on mTOR. This event permits mTOR to activate 2 p70S6 kinases known as S6 kinase 1 and 2, which, in turn, catalyze phosphorylation of S6, a 40S ribosomal protein required to drive messenger RNA (mRNA) translation and protein synthesis. In addition, through a separate pathway, mTOR activates the eukaryotic initiation factor 4E, which is also necessary for mRNA translation and ribosomal biosynthesis. Thus, mTOR plays a critical role in regulation of protein synthesis and cell cycle progression from late G1 into S phase. Logically, then, blockade of mTOR by sirolimus inhibits mRNA translation and protein synthesis and arrests T-cell cycle progression to S phase. Everolimus has the same mechanism of action but has a shorter half-life.[25–27]

THE ANTIMETABOLIC AGENTS

Mechanistically, mycophenolic acid (MPA) is an antimetabolite and acts at the S phase of cell cycle progression by interfering with purine synthesis. MPA interferes with the de novo pathway of purine biosynthesis by preventing the conversion of inosine monophosphate to xanthine monophosphate. MPA is a selective, reversibly noncompetitive inhibitor of inosine monophosphate dehydrogenase, the rate-limiting enzyme in de novo purine synthesis. This inhibition results in intracellular depletion of guanosine nucleotides, thereby halting the progression of activated T and B cells during the S phase of the cell cycle.[28,29]

Two major cellular pathways are involved in purine synthesis: the de novo pathway and the salvage pathway. Because T and B lymphocytes are critically dependent for their proliferation on de novo synthesis of purines, whereas other cell types can use salvage pathways, MPA has a potent cytostatic effect on lymphocytes.

CORTICOSTEROIDS

Corticosteroids exert a variety of actions, but those most important to transplantation include the disruption of APC functions and inhibition of proinflammatory cytokine synthesis. Corticosteroids also cause a profound but transient lymphopenia, particularly of the T-cell population. This situation is because of a redistribution of cells out of the intravascular and into the extravascular lymphoid compartment. This particular effect is typically observed with high-dose administration of steroids used for induction immunotherapy or treatment of acute rejection and is not expected with maintenance doses of steroids. Glucocorticoids have an immunosuppressive effect on proinflammatory T cells, whereas they stimulate regulatory T-cell activity **Fig. 2**.[30,31]

BELATACEPT

Belatacept is the most recent addition to the maintenance immunosuppression regimens and differs from traditional maintenance drugs in that it is a fusion protein composed of the Fc fragment of a human IgG1 immunoglobulin linked to the extracellular domain of CTLA-4.[32] Because CTLA-4 is a molecule crucial for T-cell costimulation, belatacept can selectively block the process of T-cell activation. Belatacept is

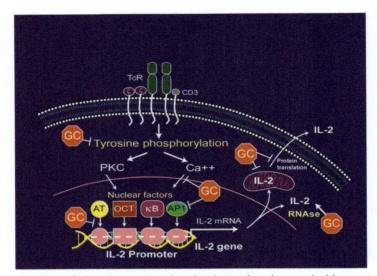

Fig. 2. On binding of the glucocorticoid molecule to the glucocorticoid receptor in the cytoplasm, the complex is then translocated to the nucleus. Once in the nucleus, the gluco-corticoid receptor binds to promoter sites of genes susceptible to glucocorticoid regulation. This situation may result in either enhancement or suppression of gene transcription. AP1, activator protein 1; AT, activated T-cell); GC, glucocorticoid; kB, Nunclear factor Kappa Beta; OCT, POU domain, class 2 transcription factor 1; PKC, protein kinase C; TcR, T-cell receptor. (*Data from* Dimitrios T, Boumpas MD, George P, et al. Glucocorticoid therapy for immune-mediated diseases: basic and clinical correlates. Ann Intern Med 1993;119(12):1198–208.)

administered intravenously and is intended to maintain graft function and limit the toxicity generated by standard immune-suppressing regimens, such as CNIs.[33,34]

THE HISTOLOGY OF GRAFT REJECTION

The pathology of transplant rejection reflects the immune mechanisms that mediate kidney allograft graft injury. Posttransplant rejection disease is now being classified based on the 2 major effector pathways; cytotoxic cells (cellular rejection) and anti-bodies (ABMR).

Acute Cell-mediated Rejection

The features of acute cell-mediated rejection are dominated by the presence of lymphocyte infiltrates in the interstitium with varying degrees of tubulitis and tubular infiltration (tubulointerstitial rejection). More severe cases can be associated with infil-tration of the blood vessels and the appearance of intimal arteritis (vascular rejection). In its most advanced form, vascular changes are associated with transmural arterial changes and extensive endothelial injury. Up to one third of allografts biopsied during clinical quiescence show some degree of interstitial inflammation and even some scattered focal tubulitis.[35] The significance of this subclinical inflammation has been debated, with conflicting evidence that these changes contribute to long-term allo-graft deterioration[36] and evidence that, at least in the short-term, this mild form of inflammation imparts no significant negative consequence on the allograft.[37] The his-tologic changes of rejection are graded by the Banff classification. In the Banff classi-fication, tubulitis is the hallmark of the diagnosis of grade I rejection, and is graded based on the number of tubules within the most inflamed area of the biopsy (**Fig. 3**).[38]

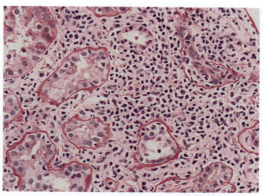

Fig. 3. Acute cellular rejection, Banff type IB. Interstitial inflammation and severe tubulitis define this type of rejection. The photomicrograph shows all grades of tubulitis.

Acute Vascular Rejection

AVR most commonly occurs in the first few months after transplantation. The detection of vascular lesions in an episode of rejection usually denotes worse prognosis and an increased chance of being resistant to standard antirejection therapy. AVR can be a manifestation of both cellular and ABMR.[39]

The histologic changes include intimal arteritis, in which lymphocytes, and monocytes (**Fig. 4**) infiltrate the vascular intima and the resulting inflammation causes intimal thickening with inflammatory cells. Besides classifying the severity of these lesions, the Banff 09 classification also added acute ABMR, which has similar vascular lesions but with associated circulatory antidonor antibody and C4d positivity in peritubular capillaries.[40]

Inflammation of the blood vessels in renal glomeruli (acute glomerulitis) can also be seen in rejection. Acute glomerulitis is characterized by the presence of mononuclear cell infiltrates and endothelial injury and swelling. Less common with acute cell mediated rejection, acute glomerulitis should always lead to the suspicion of ABMR,

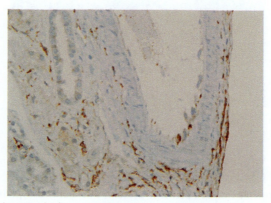

Fig. 4. AVR; the micrograph shows CD68-positive monocytes in the superficial vascular intima characteristic of mild intimal arteritis (ie, mild vascular rejection).

particularly in cases with minimal vascular involvement, or those with polymorphonu-clear leukocyte within the glomerular capillaries. The presence of donor-specific antibody and of C4d staining can usually differentiate cellular AVR and acute ABMR.

Antibody-Mediated Rejection

The immunologic mechanisms driving the development of acute ABMR occur in response to donor class I or class II alloantigens, which are particularly well expressed on activated endothelial cells. Antigens or antigenic determinants are carried by APCs to peripheral lymphoid organs where they are recognized by β cells. B cells differentiate into naive plasma cells that can secret antidonor-specific antibodies.[41] Alternatively, an-tigens may be presented locally in the allograft and induce antibody production inde-pendent of lymphoid tissue. Although the latter has not been confirmed, it seems like the result is secretion of immunoglobulin with T-cell help.[42]

Antibody deposition on vascular endothelial cells leads to in situ antigen-antibody interaction, with activation of the complement cascade. Deposition of activated com-plement results in activation of complement receptor-mediated neutrophil and macro-phage chemotaxis, cytolysis, and apoptosis of target cells, including endothelial cells. Other changes include vasospasm through the release of prostaglandin from macro-phages, edema through histamine release, and intravascular thrombosis through the triggering of endothelial synthesis of procoagulants and tissue factors. Several renal changes are characteristic for ABMR but none is pathognomonic. The 2003 Banff classification defined the criteria for diagnosing ABMR by 3 essential aspects, including (1) the presence of morphologic evidence of acute tissue injury, such as acute tubular injury, neutrophils, and/or mononuclear cells within the peritubular cap-illaries or glomerulus, and/or glomerular thrombosis, intimal arteritis, fibrinoid necrosis with or without transmural inflammation in the arteries; (2) the presence of immuno-pathologic evidence of antibody activity such as intense C4d in peritubular capillaries (>50% of capillaries) (**Fig. 5**); and (3) serologic evidence of circulating antibodies against HLA antigen or other donor-specific antigens. The C4d deposition should be diffuse and intense to diagnose ABMR (>50% of the peritubular capillaries). The presence and margination of inflammatory cells, particularly polymorphonuclear neu-trophils, and mononuclear cells.[38]

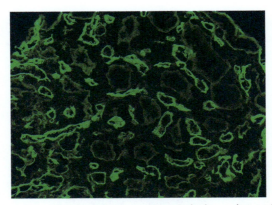

Fig. 5. Diffuse deposition of complement protein C4d along the peritubular capillaries shown by direct immunofluorescence testing. Deposition of C4d is one of the diagnostic criteria used to establish ABMR.

Immunosuppressant Nephrotoxicity

Although there are a variety of protocols for calcineurin minimization, conversion, and elimination, most immune suppression protocols still use a CNI. Acute calcineurin renal toxicity is related to afferent arteriolar vasoconstriction, leading to reduced renal blood flow and tubular ischemia. In addition, FK506 (Prograf) has direct glomerular constrictive effect. Although toxicity of both calcineurins is dose dependent, nephrotoxicity can occur in 15% to 20% of patients receiving lower doses of these drugs, particularly in those receiving FK506. Acute nephrotoxicity is uncommon in modern kidney transplant cases because of the introduction of these drugs in lower doses. Lesions of acute toxicity are seen more often in native kidney biopsies of recipients of other organ transplants. The earliest feature in these biopsies is reversible isometric tubular epithelial vacuolization and acute tubular injury, and/or arteriolar hyalinosis. Less commonly, biopsies may have features of thrombotic microangiopathy, which has also been reported with the mTOR inhibitor sirolimus. Sirolimus tubulopathy is associated with induction of tubular and podocyte apoptosis, particularly in grafts with delayed graft function, and presents with obstructive intratubular casts surrounded by regenerating tubular epithelium and tubular dilatations.

BK Nephropathy

BK virus was first described in immune-suppressed kidney transplant recipients in the early 1970s. The early reports documented that the virus resided within the transitional urothelium and was shed by more than 65% of immune-suppressed transplant recipients. Almost 2 decades later, infection of the renal parenchyma by BK virus was reported and polyoma virus–associated nephropathy (PVAN) has become one of the major challenges of clinical transplantation. The rapid increase in number of cases in the early 2000s has been attributed to increased potency of immune suppression and to the increased rates of transplantation of diabetics and older patients. The inability to expand BK-specific T cells in heavily immune-suppressed patients is believed to precipitate active infection. Viral replication in the renal parenchyma results in cytopathic changes that cause tubular apoptosis and inflammatory infiltration and lead to tubular cell injury. Alternatively, viral replication may activate adaptive immunity to perpetuate injury and cause tubular cell injury and cell death. Tubular destruction is usually followed by fibrosis and scarring, loss of kidney function, and kidney loss.

The diagnosis of BK nephropathy is based on the presence of characteristic interstitial inflammation in the deep cortex and medulla, which spares the superficial cortex. Distinguishing features include the presence of various viral inclusions in the tubules, mostly large inclusions with enlarged coarsely vesicular nuclei, and by the less frequent presence of decoy cells, which are large intranuclear acidophilic inclusions rimmed by a ring of dense chromatin at the nuclear membrane. Tubular injury is manifested by the presence of acute tubular necrosis, with sloughing cells and accumulation of coarsely granular debris in tubular lumens.[43] There is no known treatment of BK viral nephropathy, except for withdrawal or reduction of immunosuppression. Other antiviral agents are usually attempted in cases without rapid response to immunosuppression reduction; these include treatment with cidofovir and leflunamide. Follow-up biopsies are usually required for patient follow-up because fluctuations in renal function as immune suppression is being reduced raise the possibility of acute rejection. Another reason is to follow the resolution of BK nephropathy in response to immune-suppression reduction and to prevent unnecessary further withdrawal of immune suppression when the nephropathy is already revolving.[44] Our observation in series of patients with repeat renal biopsies has indicated that regardless of the PVAN status, there is almost always an increase in the Banff chronic score, and progression of interstitial fibrosis. This finding has stimulated our team to adopt prospective monitoring to diagnose early the viral infection and intervene before the onset of tubulointerstitial nephritis and renal fibrosis.[45,46]

Chronic Allograft Changes

Renal allografts undergo gradual, cumulative, and incremental damage to the nephron from time-dependent immunologic and nonimmunologic causes.[47] In early classifications, the chronic pathologic changes were called chronic rejection,[48] chronic transplant nephropathy,[49] and chronic allograft nephropathy (CAN).[50] The constellation of histologic findings of arteriosclerosis and arteriosclerosis, glomerulosclerosis, tubular atrophy, and interstitial fibrosis with chronic inflammation are seen in most allografts with chronic injury and are largely similar to chronic kidney disease (CKD) in the native kidney, regardless of the cause.[51] Because most of the histopathologic features of CKD in the allograft could not be specifically attributed to an allospecific response (chronic rejection, CAN) was adopted for the Banff working classification.[50] Chronic allograft injury is clinically characterized by progressive deterioration of graft function, proteinuria, and hypertension.[52]

Chronic ABMR is diagnosed when interstitial fibrosis and tubular atrophy are associated with 1 or more of these features: chronic transplant glomerulopathy, chronic microvascular injury, intragraft deposition of C4d, and the presence of donor-specific antibody.[40] Chronic T-cell–mediated rejection is suspected in grafts that show tubulitis along with thickening of the elastic layer of the blood vessels, fibrous intimal hyperplasia, and variable inflammation in the intima, which are all features of chronic transplant vasculopathy. A long list of non–immune-mediated conditions can also cause chronic allograft injury or exacerbate an immune injury. Causes of nonimmune chronic allograft injury include donor factors such as senescence, nephrosclerosis, donor vasculopathy, or recipient diseases such as hypertension, diabetes, and hyperlipidemia (the metabolic syndrome). Other nonimmune causes include exposure to nephrotoxins, viral infections, and reflux nephropathy.[52–54] A subset of allografts show chronic transplant glomerulopathy, possibly a form of allograft rejection.[55,56]

REFERENCES

1. Auchincloss H Jr, Sultan H. Antigen processing and presentation in transplantation. Curr Opin Immunol 1996;8:681–7.
2. Hall BM. Cells mediating allograft rejection. Transplantation 1991;51:1141–51.
3. Land W, Schneeberger H, Schleibner S, et al. The beneficial effect of human recombinant superoxide dismutase on acute and chronic rejection events in recipients of cadaveric renal transplants. Transplantation 1994;57(2):211–7.
4. Land W. The potential impact of the reperfusion injury on acute and chronic rejection events following organ transplantation. Transplant Proc 1994;26(6):3169–71.
5. Land W. Innate alloimmunity: history and current knowledge. Exp Clin Transplant 2001;5(1):575–84.
6. Liu W, Li XC. An overview on non-T cell pathways in transplant rejection and tolerance. Curr Opin Organ Transplant 2010;15(4):422–6.
7. Yu G, Xu X, Vu MD, et al. NK cells promote transplant tolerance by killing donor antigen-presenting cells. J Exp Med 2006;203:1851–8.

8. Zhou X, Bailey-Bucktrout S, Jeker LT, et al. Plasticity of CD4+Foxp3+ T cells. Curr Opin Immunol 2009;21:281–5.

9. Heeger PS, Dinavahi R. Transplant immunology for non-immunologist. Mt Sinai J Med 2012;79(3):376–87.

10. Bloom D, Chang Z, Pauly K, et al. BAFF is increased in renal transplant patients following treatment with alemtuzumab. Am J Transplant 2009;9:1835–45.

11. Kwun J, Bulut P, Kim E, et al. The role of B cells in solid organ transplantation. Semin Immunol 2012;24(2):96–108.

12. Stegall MD, Chedid MF, Cornell LD. The role of complement in antibody-mediated rejection in kidney transplantation. Nat Rev Nephrol 2012;8(11):670–8.

13. Delves PJ, Roitt IM. The immune system. Second of two parts. N Engl J Med 2000;343(2):108–17.

14. Guttmann RD, Soulillou JP, Moore LW, et al. Proposed consensus for definitions and endpoints for clinical trials of acute kidney transplant rejection. Am J Kidney Dis 1998;31(6 Suppl 1):S40–6.

15. Gaber LW, Moore LW, Gaber AO, et al. Utility of standardized histological classification in the management of acute rejection. 1995 Efficacy Endpoints Conference. Transplantation 1998;65(3):376–80 [Erratum appears in Transplantation 1998;66(8):1121].

16. Gaber LW, Gaber AO, Vera SR, et al. Successful reversal of hyperacute renal allograft rejection with the anti-CD3 monoclonal OKT3. Transplantation 1992;54(5):930–2.

17. Gaber AO, Monaco AP, Russell JA, et al. Rabbit antithymocyte globulin (thymoglobulin): 25 years and new frontiers in solid organ transplantation and haematology. Drugs 2010;70(6):691–732.

18. Gaber AO, Knight RJ, Patel S, et al. A review of the evidence for use of thymoglobulin induction in renal transplantation. Transplant Proc 2010;42(5):1395–400.

19. Weaver TA, Kirk AD. Alemtuzumab. Transplantation 2007;84:1545–7.

20. Tydén G, Ekberg H, Tufveson G, et al. A randomized, double-blind, placebo-controlled study of single dose rituximab as induction in renal transplantation: a 3-year follow-up. Transplantation 2012;94(3):e21–2.

21. Epifanova OI. Mechanisms underlying the differential sensitivity of proliferating and resting cells to external factors. Int Rev Cytol Suppl 1977;(5):303–35.

22. Crossen PE, Morgan WF. Analysis of human lymphocyte cell cycle time in culture measured by sister chromatid differential staining. Exp Cell Res 1977;104(2):453–7.

23. Tilney NL, Strom TB, Paul LC, editors. Transplantation biology: cellular and molecular aspects. Philadelphia: Lippincott-Raven; 1996. p. 657–71.

24. Coico R, Sunshine G, Benjamini E, editors. Immunology: a short course. Hoboken (NJ): John Wiley; 2003. p. 129–47.

25. Hay N, Sonenberg N. Upstream and downstream of mTOR. Genes Dev 2004;18:1926.

26. Koehl GE, Schlitt HJ, Geissler EK. Rapamycin and tumor growth: mechanisms behind its anticancer activity. Transplant Rev 2005;19:20.

27. Lisik W, Kahan BD. Proliferation signal inhibitors: chemical, biologic, and clinical properties. Transplant Rev 2005;19:186.

28. Sollinger HW. Mycophenolates in transplantation. Clin Transplant 2004;18:485.

29. Franklin TJ, Cook JM. The inhibition of nucleic acid synthesis by mycophenolic acid. Biochem J 1969;113:515.

30. Zen M, Canova M, Campana C, et al. The kaleidoscope of glucorticoid effects on immune system. Autoimmun Rev 2011;10(6):305–10.
31. Boumpas DT, Chrousos GP, Wilder RL, et al. Glucocorticoid therapy for immune-mediated diseases: basic and clinical correlates. Ann Intern Med 1993;119:1198.
32. Yabu JM, Vincenti F. Novel immunosuppression: small molecules and biologics. Semin Nephrol 2007;27(4):479–86.
33. Vincenti F, Larsen C, Durrbach A, et al. Costimulation blockade with belatacept in renal transplantation. N Engl J Med 2005;353(8):770–81.
34. Larsen CP, Grinyó J, Medina-Pestana J, et al. Belatacept-based regimens versus a cyclosporine A-based regimen in kidney transplant recipients: 2-year results from the BENEFIT and BENEFT-EXT studies. Transplantation 2010;90:1528–35.
35. Buchmann TN, Wolff T, Bachmann A, et al. Repeat true surveillance biopsies in kidney transplantation. Transplantation 2012;93:908–13.
36. Rush DN, Nickerson P, Gough J, et al. Beneficial effects of treatment of early subclinical rejection: a randomized study. J Am Soc Nephrol 1998;9:2129–34.
37. Nankivell BJ, Chapman JR. The significance of subclinical rejection and the value of protocol biopsies. Am J Transplant 2006;6(9):2006–12.
38. Racusen LC, Halloran PF, Solez K. Banff 2003 meeting report: new diagnostic insights and standards. Am J Transplant 2004;4(10):1562–6.
39. Gaber L, Croker B. Pathology of kidney and pancreas transplantation. In: Srinivas TR, Shoskes D, editors. Kidney and pancreas transplantation practical guide. New York: Humana Press; 2011. p. 111–38.
40. Sis B, Mengel M, Haas M, et al. Banff '09 meeting report: antibody mediated graft deterioration and implementation of Banff working groups. Am J Transplant 2010;10(3):464–71.
41. Truong LD, Barrios R, Adrogue HE, et al. Acute antibody-mediated rejection of renal transplant: pathogenetic and diagnostic considerations. Arch Pathol Lab Med 2007;131(8):1200–8.
42. Cai J, Terasaki PI. Humoral theory of transplantation: mechanism, prevention, and treatment. Hum Immunol 2005;66(4):334–42.
43. Drachenberg CB, Hirsch HH, Ramos E, et al. Polyomavirus disease in renal transplantation: review of pathological findings and diagnostic methods. Hum Pathol 2005;36(12):1245–55.
44. Ramos E, Drachenberg CB, Wali R, et al. The decade of polyomavirus BK-associated nephropathy: state of affairs. Transplantation 2009;87(5):621–30.
45. Gaber LW, Egidi MF, Stratta RJ, et al. Clinical utility of histological features of polyomavirus allograft nephropathy. Transplantation 2006;82(2):196–204.
46. Knight RJ, Gaber LW, Patel SJ, et al. Screening for BK viremia reduces but does not eliminate the risk of BK nephropathy: a single-center retrospective analysis. Transplantation 2013;95(7):949–54.
47. Nankivell BJ, Borrows RJ, Fung CL, et al. The natural history of chronic allograft nephropathy. N Engl J Med 2003;349(24):2326–33.
48. Zollingerh HU, Mihatch MJ. Renal pathology in biopsy: light, electron and immunofluorescent microscopy, and clinical aspects. New York: Springer-Verlag; 1978.
49. Croker B, Ramos EL. Pathology of the renal allograft. In: Tischer C, Brenner BM, editors. Renal pathology with clinical and functional correlations. Philadelphia: Lippincott; 1994.
50. Solez K, Axelsen RA, Benediktsson H, et al. International standardization of criteria for the histologic diagnosis of renal allograft rejection: the Banff working classification of kidney transplant pathology. Kidney Int 1993;44(2):411–22.

51. Heptinstall R. Pathology of the kidney. Boston: Little Brown; 1974.
52. Chan L, Wiseman A, Wang W, et al. Outcomes and complications of renal transplantation. In: Schrier R, editor. Diseases of the kidney and urinary tract. Philadelphia: Lippincott Williams & Wilkins; 2007.
53. Chapman JR. Longitudinal analysis of chronic allograft nephropathy: clinicopathologic correlations. Kidney Int Suppl 2005;(99):S108–12.
54. Kasiske BL, Gaston RS, Gourishankar S, et al. Long term deterioration of kidney allograft function. Am J Transplant 2005;5(6):1405–14.
55. Gloor JM, Sethi S, Stegall MD, et al. Transplant glomerulopathy: subclinical incidence and association with alloantibody. Am J Transplant 2007;7(9):2124–32.
56. Cosio FG, Gloor JM, Sethi S, et al. Transplant glomerulopathy. Am J Transplant 2008;8(3):492–6.

Robotic-Assisted Kidney Transplantation

Ivo Tzvetanov, MD[a],*, Pier C. Giulianotti, MD[b],
Lorena Bejarano-Pineda, MD[a], Hoonbae Jeon, MD[a],
Raquel Garcia-Roca, MD[a], Francesco Bianco, MD[b],
José Oberholzer, MD[a], Enrico Benedetti, MD[a]

KEYWORDS

- Robotic surgery • Kidney transplant • Obesity

KEY POINTS

- Minimally invasive surgery has revolutionized general surgery. Robotic-assisted surgery has presented an opportunity to perform organ transplantation in a minimally invasive fashion.
- Kidney transplantation is the best treatment of patients with chronic renal failure. About two-thirds of kidney transplant recipients have a body mass index of 25 kg/m^2 or greater. This finding implies an increased risk of complications and poorer outcomes.
- The major advantage of minimally invasive surgical technology in the form of robotic surgery is reduction of difficulties associated with kidney transplantation for obese patients.
- Benefits such as reduced recovery period and significantly reduced number of wound complications such as surgical site infections have been attained with the robotic surgical approach.
- More than 70 robotic-assisted kidney transplants have been performed successfully. Most of the recipients have experienced excellent outcomes in the short-term. The initial results have shown the feasibility of the technique in transplantation.
- From our experience, we believe that robotic-assisted surgery has expanded the ability to complete complex surgical procedures in a minimally invasive fashion. However, advanced training and experience are required in all surgeons who are interested in pursuing this technique.

The authors declare no funding or conflicts of interest.
[a] Division of Transplantation, Department of Surgery, University of Illinois at Chicago, 840 South Wood Street, CSB 402 (MC 958), Chicago, IL 60612, USA; [b] Division of Minimally Invasive and Robotic Surgery, Department of Surgery, University of Illinois at Chicago, 840 South Wood Street, CSB 435E (MC 958), Chicago, IL 60612, USA
* Corresponding author.
E-mail address: itzveta@uic.edu

Surg Clin N Am 93 (2013) 1309–1323
http://dx.doi.org/10.1016/j.suc.2013.08.003
0039-6109/13/$ – see front matter © 2013 Elsevier Inc. All rights reserved.

surgical.theclinics.com

The introduction of minimally invasive and precise surgical robotic systems, such as the Da Vinci surgical system (Intuitive Surgical), has expanded the possibility of performing more difficult surgeries and has shown promise in organ transplantation. Minimally invasive surgical technologies have shown significant benefits, such as reduced recovery period, fewer wound complications, and reduced surgical scars. Robotic surgery has been successfully used in kidney and pancreas transplantation,[1] and donor hepatectomy for living donor (LD) liver transplantation.[2]

Kidney transplantation is the best treatment of patients with end-stage renal disease (ESRD). Obesity is a common comorbidity among potential kidney transplant recipients in the United States,[3] causing longer wait times on the waiting list for kidney transplantation for obese patients compared with nonobese patients. Approximately two-thirds of kidney transplant recipients have a body mass index (BMI, calculated as weight in kilograms divided by the square of height in meters) of 25 kg/m^2 or greater, which implicates a higher risk of complications such as delayed graft function, surgical site infection (SSI) and episodes of acute rejection.[4] According to Lynch and colleagues,[5] SSI is significantly associated with graft loss and a tendency toward an inferior rate of patient survival. However, obese recipients who avoid SSI have outcomes similar to nonobese recipients (**Fig. 1**).

Considering the negative impact of obesity on outcomes and its increased risk of complications, many surgical centers are skeptical about listing morbidly obese patients for renal transplantation. Therefore, one of the goals with this new surgical approach is to minimize the difficulties associated with kidney transplantation for obese patients with ESRD.[6]

SELECTION AND PRETRANSPLANT EVALUATION

Renal transplantation is the most effective form of renal replacement. However, the number of available organ remains limited, whereas the number of patients with

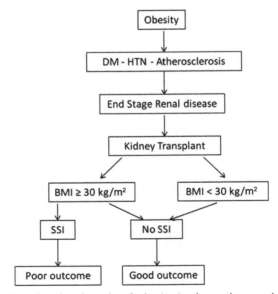

Fig. 1. Proposed algorithm for the role of obesity in the pathogenesis of ESRD and the outcome of transplant recipients. DM, diabetes mellitus; HTN, hypertension.

ESRD keeps increasing. The primary goals of pretransplant evaluation are to assess overall risk and to identify modifiable risk, so as to optimize successful transplant outcomes and to better educate the prospective recipients and close relatives concerning all aspects, of the transplant process, along with all known and potential risks (**Fig. 2**). The transplant team should anticipate a prospective recipient's individualized problems and risks and, accordingly, make a plan to address any potential surgical and postsurgical situations.

The best time to refer a patient for transplant evaluation is when their glomerular filtration rate (GFR) is within the range of 15 to 30 mL/min/1.73 m^2 or when the patient has chronic kidney disease (CKD) stage 4.[7] Further, in the United States, patients need to be counseled that, for them to commence accruing wait time on the United Network for Organ Sharing waiting list, they must have an estimated GFR of 20 mL/min or less.

Special Considerations

Age

There is no age limit for kidney transplantation; however, access to transplantation should be for those patients who have a life expectancy of longer than 1 year.[8]

Malignancy

An active tumor is an absolute contraindication to transplantation. **Box 1** summarizes major contraindications for renal transplantation. A cancer with a high chance of recurrence is also a general contraindication for LD transplantation. The rationale for these contraindications is that the prevalence of cancer is significantly higher in transplant recipients compared with patients who remain in dialysis.[9] For most cancers, a disease-free interval of 2 to 5 years after a documented cure is appropriate to reduce the risk of cancer recurrence. However, the decision to list a patient with a history of malignancy needs to be individualized, taking into account the prognosis of the particular tumor.[10]

Infectious disease

Patients with hepatitis B and C are acceptable candidates for kidney transplantation, if they do not have cirrhotic changes in liver biopsy.[11] In addition, patients positive for human immunodeficiency virus with a controlled viral load are no longer

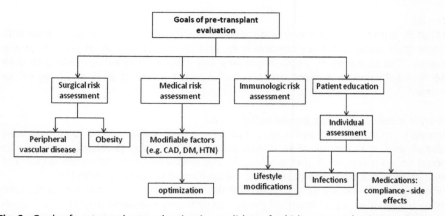

Fig. 2. Goals of pretransplant evaluation in candidates for kidney transplantation. CAD, coronary artery disease; DM, diabetes mellitus; HTN, hypertension.

Box 1
Major contraindications to kidney transplantation

Reversible kidney disease

Active neoplasm

Severe lung or cardiovascular disease

Severe cirrhosis biopsy proven

Patient nonadherent to medications

Active substance abuse or uncontrolled psychiatric disorders

Current infection

Life expectancy of less than 1 year

---

contraindicated for renal transplantation. Cytomegalovirus (CMV) remains the most significant and prevalent posttransplant infection, and therefore recipients should receive prophylaxis after transplantation.[11]

Coronary artery disease

Individuals at high risk for coronary artery disease (CAD) should be assessed and screened. Initial screening can be performed by noninvasive tests, such as the dobutamine stress test. However, patients with positive tests should be considered for revascularization before transplant surgery.[12] CAD is the leading cause of death after renal transplantation.[13]

Immunologic risk

Prospective recipients should have screening tests conducted to detect preformed HLA antibodies. Patients with one of the following characteristics are considered at high risk for rejection: (1) African American; (2) retransplant (if the first transplant failed because of rejection); (3) recipient with panel reactive antibody (PRA) >10/%; (4) ABO incompatible; and (5) positive cross-match. Being ABO incompatible is no longer a contraindication for LD transplantation; however, such patients should receive desensitizing therapy in order to decrease antibody titers.

Obesity

BMI of 30 kg/m^2 or greater is an independent risk for SSI,[5] which is associated with poorer graft survival, longer hospital stay, and an increased risk of cardiovascular disease. The evidence to exclude patients from the waiting list according to their BMI is insufficient, but most centers use a cutoff value of BMI of 40 kg/m^2 or greater.[8]

Lifestyle modification and psychosocial issues

Cigarette smoking has been associated with an increased risk of cardiovascular disease and malignancy after transplantation. Therefore, prospective recipients should be encouraged to quit smoking.[14] The presence of an adequate social and psychological support system needs to be confirmed for patients with CKD.[15]

Preemptive LD kidney transplantation is the best option for anyone with advanced kidney failure. Also, a pretransplant evaluation provides a valuable opportunity to evaluate the patient's expectations, assess risk, and implement controls for modifiable risk factors that are associated with adverse outcomes.

SURGICAL APPROACH

Once a successful pretransplant evaluation has been attained, the patient is presented to the transplant interdisciplinary team. Because longer time on hemodialysis has a negative impact on posttransplant outcomes, the goal is to perform kidney transplant as soon as possible.[16] Once a suitable LD becomes available for a patient who is an LD candidate, the surgical approach depends on the patient's BMI. If the patient has a BMI less than 30 kg/m^2, an open surgical approach is chosen. Otherwise, if the patient is obese, with a BMI of 30 kg/m^2 or greater, the patient is approached by a minimally invasive robotic-assisted technique. Patients who do not have potential LD are placed on the waiting list. During the waiting time, patients with BMI of 30 kg/m^2 or greater start simultaneously a weight loss program. Once a deceased donor becomes available, obese patients undergo robotic-assisted transplantation and nonobese patients undergo open surgery (**Fig. 3**). Previous surgeries are not considered a contraindication to perform a robotic-assisted procedure. The only exclusion criteria are severe atherosclerosis of the iliac vessels in the recipient and the graft vessels (for a deceased donor).

After a patient is scheduled for elective LD kidney transplantation, preoperative planning and procedures may take up to 1 or 2 weeks, depending on the patient's immunologic risk. Patients who have positive cross-match or are ABO incompatible with their donors need to undergo desensitization, which includes plasmapheresis before surgery, in order to decrease the titers of the reactive antibodies. Our opinion is that obese patients with high immunologic risk are excellent candidates for a minimally invasive surgical approach, because their immunosuppressive protocol is more aggressive, and prevention of surgical complications becomes extremely important.

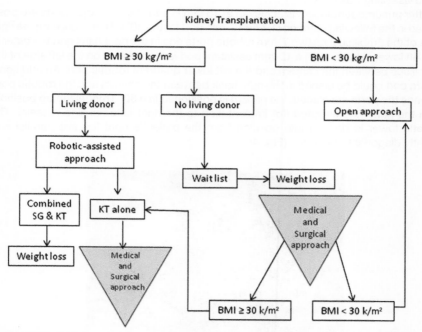

Fig. 3. Surgical approach of the kidney transplant candidate. KT, kidney transplant; SG, surgery.

The patients are admitted to the transplant unit the day before the surgery, with no oral intake for at least 6 to 8 hours.

SURGICAL PROCEDURE
Backbench Preparation of the Graft

This step of the procedure has some differences from the original graft preparation for open transplantation. The purpose is to facilitate orientation of the organ before the vascular anastomosis is started and to minimize bleeding from the surface of the kidney after the reperfusion. Regardless of the origin of the kidney graft, LD or deceased donor, backbench preparation for robotic implantation follows some specific steps. The adipose capsule is meticulously legated with 3-0 silk during excision. Renal vein and artery are dissected toward the hilum and marked with marking pen, depending on the site of implantation, right or left. The ureter is appropriately shortened and speculated.

Patient Positioning and Port Placement

After induction of general anesthesia, a 3-way Foley catheter is placed. This strategy allows filling the bladder with 100 to 150 mL of diluted methylene blue solution after completion of the vascular anastomosis, which facilitates identification of the bladder and prevents spatial interference during the vascular suturing.

The patient is positioned supine, with parted and flexed legs; shoulder block and tape were used to avoid the patient sliding during the operation. After the patient is prepared in the sterile fashion, a 7-cm midline incision approximately 5 cm below the xyphoid process is made and a hand access device is placed. Depending on the body habitus of the recipient, the location of this midline incision could be closer to the umbilicus in order to allow easier access to the surgical field for the bedside hand-assisting cosurgeon.

After pneumoperitoneum is achieved at 15 mm Hg, the laparoscopic ports are positioned in the following manner: (1) one 12-mm port for the 30° robotic scope on the right side of the umbilicus; (2) two 7-mm robotic ports one in the right flank and the other in the left lower quadrant; (3) a 12-mm assistant port is then placed on the left side of the umbilicus between the camera and the left lower quadrant robotic port. An additional 5-mm port could be placed in the right flank between the camera and the robotic port.

Once the ports are placed, the patient is positioned in a 30° Trendelenburg position, with the right side elevated (for implantation to the right external iliac vessels). The robotic tower is docked into position from the patient's right leg site parallel and slightly diagonal to the body (**Fig. 4**).

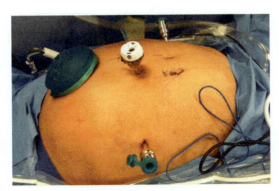

Fig. 4. Port placements in the kidney transplant recipient.

Vascular Exposure

The right colon is mobilized, and right external iliac artery and vein exposed. The iliac vessels are dissected free, using a bipolar forceps and a hook electrocautery. In order to facilitate the exposure and the dissection around the external iliac vein, a vessel loop is used to retract the artery upwards. Another vessel loop is placed around the iliac vein to allow dissection on the posterior surface of the vein. Because the iliac vessels need to be completely mobilized at least 5 cm long in case any collaterals are found, they need to be legated using Prolene 5-0 and then transected.

Graft Implantation and Reperfusion

Once the external iliac vessels are completely dissected free, 2 robotic bulldog clamps are used to occlude the external iliac vein proximal and distal (**Fig. 5**). Robotic Potts scissors are used to create a venotomy to about 15 mm (**Fig. 6**). A 12-cm, double-needle, 5-0 Gore-Tex suture with a knot in the middle is placed at the corner of the venotomy. Kidney graft is inserted in the abdominal cavity by the assisting surgeon and positioned parallel to the dissected iliac vessels. Previous marking of the renal vessels of the graft facilitates the extremely important step of initial orientation. Venovenous anastomosis is completed in an end-to-side fashion with running suture (**Fig. 7**). If needed, interrupted stitches of 5-0 Prolene are used to reinforce the anastomosis. Subsequently, the external iliac artery is clamped between robotic bulldogs, and an oval window (proportional to the size of the renal artery of the graft) is made in the anterior wall of the artery with robotic scissors. To facilitate this precise step, a 5-0 Prolene stitch is placed trough the anterior wall of the external iliac artery and gentle pulling is applied. The arterial anastomosis is completed in an end-to-side fashion with a 12-cm double-needle 6-0 Gore-Tex suture with a knot in the middle (**Fig. 8**).

Once vascular suturing is completed, venous clamps are removed first, followed by immediate removal of the arterial clamps. The reperfusion of the organ and hemostasis are verified and bleeding points secured with 6-0 Prolene suture. We routinely use a robotic fluorescence camera and intravenous injection of 3 mL indocyanine green. This strategy allows confirmation of the complete and homogeneous reperfusion of the graft. At this point, the pressure of the pneumoperitoneum is decreased

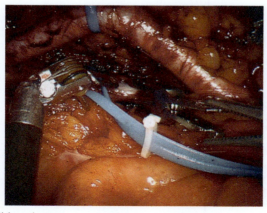

Fig. 5. Robotic bulldog clamps.

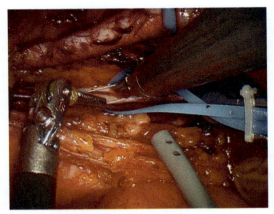

Fig. 6. Venotomy of the external iliac vein in the recipient.

to 10 mm Hg to minimize the possible negative effect of high intra-abdominal pressure on the graft perfusion.

Ureter Cystoneostomy

The urinary bladder is filled with diluted methylene blue solution in order to facilitate its identification. Distending the bladder at the beginning of the operation could cause spatial interference, especially in patients with preserved diuresis from the native kidneys. Once the dome of the bladder is localized, the muscular layers are incised and the bladder mucosa is prepared. The ureter is anastomosed to the bladder with 5-0 Monocryl running suture using typical antireflux technique, and suturing full thickness of the ureteral wall with the mucosal layer of the bladder. Utilization of a ureteral stent is optional. On completion of the anastomosis, the sero-muscular layer is closed over the ureterocystostomy with 3-0 Vycril to create an anti-reflux mechanism.

At the end of the procedure, the minilaparotomy is closed with running 0 polydioxa-none and the 2 12-mm port sites are closed from inside the abdomen with an

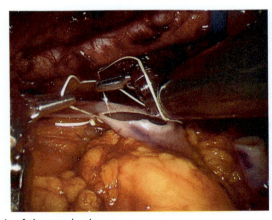

Fig. 7. Anastomosis of the renal vein.

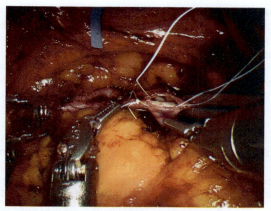

Fig. 8. Anastomosis of the renal artery.

endosuture needle and 0 Vycril suture. Skin incisions are closed cosmetically. Placement of drains is not necessary (**Fig. 9**).

IMMEDIATE POSTOPERATIVE CARE

After completion of the operation, the recipients are brought to the surgical intensive care unit, where they receive close monitoring of urine output (UOP) and arterial and central venous pressure. More than 95% of recipients experience immediate graft function and very high diuresis, which may cause volume fluctuations and electrolyte derangements. Hemogram, electrolytes, and renal function are monitored every 6 hours within the first 24 hours, and then every 12 hours. We cannot overemphasize the importance of proper fluid management. The amount of urine produced by the graft may vary widely in the early postoperative period. Within the first 24 hours, the UOP is replaced with 1:1 (mL per mL) normal saline solution, given in addition to the maintenance fluids. Because volume replacements can be high, electrolyte replacement should be performed separately. Also, avoiding graft hypoperfusion is

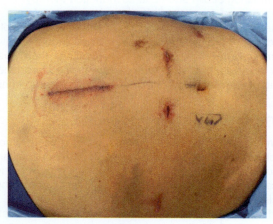

Fig. 9. Port positioning in the recipient after closure.

paramount, because this can cause the onset of acute tubular necrosis. During the next 48 hours, graft function stabilizes and fluid replacement is decreased to 50% of the UOP and to standard maintenance intravenous fluids (IVFs). Oral intake is resumed on postoperative day (POD) 1 and gradually advanced. IVFs are discontinued by POD 4. Knowledge of patient pretransplant UOP is important, because there are patients who experience daily UOP before transplantation, and this urine must be taken into account in order to achieve an appropriate assessment of posttransplant UOP.

Serum creatinine level is expected to decrease at least 50% on POD 1, which is taken in to consideration when assessing proper graft function. Signs of graft dysfunction include oligoanuria; a plateauing of or increase in serum creatinine level despite adequate intravascular volume; and blood pressure. Once the cause of graft dysfunction has been identified, it should be rectified as soon as possible to avoid deleterious outcomes. Delayed graft function, defined as the need for dialysis within the first week after transplantation, is detrimental to early and long-term graft survival. For recipients with delayed graft function and with no evident cause, it is recommended that ultrasonography and biopsy be performed every 7 to 10 days, until there is overt improvement in graft function.

As discussed earlier, recipients begin a liquid diet within postoperative 1; and, according to their tolerance of it without nausea or vomiting, are then allowed to advance to a regular diet within the next 2 to 3 days. Kidney transplant recipients have an increased risk for acute pseudo-obstruction; therefore, they receive a bowel regimen of docusate or bisacodyl from POD 1. The Foley catheter is removed on POD 4; recipients are encouraged to start pulmonary physiotherapy and early ambulation, so as to decrease the incidence of nosocomial pneumonia and deep venous thrombosis. Recipients with additional risk factors for venous thrombosis receive subcutaneous heparin or low-molecular-weight heparin.

Immunosuppressant therapy in the immediate postoperative period is based on recipient immunologic risks. All recipients receive a rapid steroid taper completed by POD 5; with the exception of positive cross-match, recipients continue receiving steroids in a low dose thereafter. Recipients also receive induction therapy, along with either rabbit antithymocyte globulin or baxiliximab, during their first few postoperative days. In addition, recipients with PRA levels greater than 30% and positive B-cell and T-cell cross-match undergo a desensitization protocol with plasmapheresis and intravenous immunoglobulin additional to induction therapy.

Patients are discharged from the hospital when they tolerate their diet, have adequate pain control via oral medication, and achieve a reasonable graft function. However, before discharge, patients and their relatives should receive a comprehensive education on the array of multiple new medications that have been initiated. Patients and their relatives also need to be aware of the importance of adherence to medications and of relevant symptoms that require follow-up consultation.

LONG-TERM POSTTRANSPLANTATION MANAGEMENT

During the first 3 months after transplant, most recipients achieve normal renal function; however, such achievement does not come about without ups and downs. Close follow-up and monitoring are mandatory to reduce the risk of nonadherence to prescribed medication, and for fostering a healthy lifestyle consisting of a good diet and regular exercise.

Recipients need to attend clinic visits 2 to 3 times a week for the first 3 weeks, then 1 to 2 times a week until POD 45. From that point onward, and until the end of the third

Table 1
Follow-up schedule

Postoperative Period	Clinic Visit
POD 1–21	2–3 times/wk
POD 22–45	1–2 times/wk
POD 45–90	Weekly
3–4 mo	Every 2–3 wk
5–6 mo	Every 3–4 wk
7–9 mo	Every 4–6 wk
10–12 mo	Every 6–8 wk
1–2 y	Every 2–4 mo
2 y onward	Every 6 mo

month, they need to attend weekly follow-up appointments (**Tables 1** and **2**). The frequency of routine follow-up clinical sessions is tailored to the personalized needs of each recipient. Follow-up clinical sessions can be executed at the outpatient clinic of the transplantation center, with the community nephrologist, or with a family practitioner with experience in posttransplantation care.

Each clinical session must include a detailed medical history and physical examination, so as to assess the state of chronic comorbidities and the possible onset of new medical conditions. The physical examination should also pay close attention to the patient's state of hydration and graft tenderness.

Laboratory tests such as a chemistry panel, complete blood count, and calcineurin inhibitor concentrations need to be performed the morning of each visit. A patient's creatinine level should be a major concern factor during each clinical visit, and the respective patient needs to be made aware of this, along with test results. An increase in a patient's creatinine level of more than 25% higher than the previous level, or a decrease in UOP, demands further investigation. The first step is to perform Doppler

Table 2
Robotic kidney transplant and control patient characteristics

Characteristics	Recipients (N = 70)
Age (y), mean (SD)	46.8 (11.8)
Gender (male), number (%)	34 (47.9)
Race (African American/Hispanic/white/other), number (%)	32/18/17/3 (46/26/24/4)
BMI (kg/m^2), mean (SD)	43 (7.1)
Dialysis, number (%)	50 (70.4)
LD, number (%)	64 (90.1)
Cold ischemia time (h; n = 68/70), mean (SD)	3.6 (5)
Warm ischemia time (min; n = 68/70), mean (SD)	52.3 (12.2)
SSIs, number (%)	0 (0)
Delayed graft function, number (%)	3 (4.2)
Creatinine at discharge (mg/dL), mean (SD)	1.8 (1.1)
Graft failure, number (%)	1 (1.4)
Deaths, number (%)	2 (2.8)

Abbreviation: SD, standard deviation.

ultrasonography to exclude structural problems in vascular vessels and the drainage system. After being addressed, the next step is to ensure an adequate state of hydration and to rule out the presence of calcineurin inhibitor toxicity. In case none is present, then performing a biopsy is the most appropriate follow-up action (**Fig. 10**).

Considering the intraperitoneal location of the graft in robotic recipients, we prefer to perform the biopsy by laparoscopic guidance. Ultrasound-guided biopsy can cause significant bleeding. The procedure is completed under general anesthesia, and antibiotic prophylaxis is routinely given. Our preference for port positioning is one infraumbilical and one in the upper quadrant on the site of the graft. Nevertheless, a single port approach is also possible. A kidney graft is visualized in the iliac fossa. A Tru-Cut biopsy needle, usually 18 G, is introduced through the abdominal wall and directed toward the upper pole of the graft. Two or 3 passages are made until a reliable specimen is obtained and verified by a pathologist. Bleeding from biopsy sites is controlled with cauterization through the second port. Ports are removed and port sites closed in standard fashion.

The patient is observed for 2 hours and discharged home. Possible complications are the same as with percutaneous biopsy. The laparoscopic guidance allows targeting the upper pole of the graft to where the likelihood of complications is significantly lower.

Cardiovascular disease, cancer, and infections are the leading causes of death in the late posttransplant period, and immunosuppression plays a major role in the pathogenesis of these complications. However, most recipients reject the graft if immunosuppression is completely withdrawn; therefore, in order to decrease the chance of complications from setting in, recipients should continue receiving the minimal amount of immunosuppressant that prevents rejection. This minimal amount should be personalized and tailored to address the unique needs of each recipient; the only way to achieve this is via close monitoring of each recipient's prescribed medications and preclinic test results during each clinic visit.

Maintenance immunosuppressive therapy includes a combination of tacrolimus and mycophenolic acid. Hispanic recipients with low risk of rejection receive cyclosporine

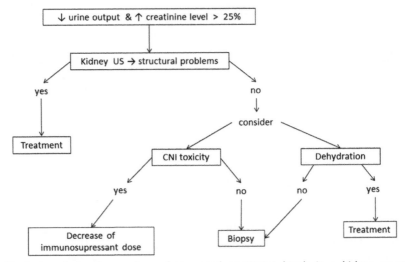

Fig. 10. Approach to the workup of increased creatinine levels in a kidney transplant recipient.

instead of tacrolimus. Antimicrobial prophylaxis consists of valganciclovir for CMV and Epstein-Barr virus; sulfamethoxazole/trimethoprim for urinary tract infection and *Pneumocystis jiroveci* pneumonia during 6 months after transplantation.

Weight gain for postkidney transplantations affects 50% to 90% of kidney transplant recipients.[17] Hyperphagia alongside recipient-associated sense of liberation from previous dietary limitations contributes to the propensity for weight gain after transplantation. The management of obesity includes behavior modification, an exercise program, and nutritional counseling. If this medical and mediational approach fails after 6 months, bariatric surgery should be considered for respective morbidly obese patients.

Encouraging a healthy lifestyle and follow-through on strategies to prevent common comorbidities should be an integral component of the individualized therapeutic regimen in renal transplanted patients. Regular exercise may help to minimize post-transplantation weight gain and might be considered important for patients with metabolic syndrome and high risk of cardiovascular disease. Obesity can otherwise contribute significantly to the development or exacerbation of common comorbidities, such as dyslipidemia, hypertension, and diabetes mellitus, in transplanted patients.[18]

CLINICAL RESULTS IN THE LITERATURE

The first fully robotic-assisted kidney transplant for an obese recipient was performed in August, 2009 and reported by Giulianotti and colleagues[19] in early 2010. It was performed in an obese 29-year-old woman with ESRD secondary to congenital obstructive uropathy. Within the same year, Boggi and colleagues[20] published the first case performed in Europe. However, the surgical technique described by Boggi and colleagues differs from ours in a few steps. The site of the incision performed in their report was a suprapubic incision (Pfannenstiel incision), and the location of the graft was retroperitoneal. Some of the advantages of our technique are facilitating handling the graft during the vascular anastomosis by hand assistance, and gaining full access to iliac vessels, especially in obese recipients. According to our experience, a periumbilical incision and positioning the graft intraperitoneally is a feasible approach, with advantages over the other technique in obese patients.

Within the last 4 years, we have applied this standardized technique to more than 70 robotic-assisted kidney transplants in obese recipients. The highest BMI of a transplanted patient was 58 kg/m^2, and the mean BMI of the group was 43 kg/m^2. In this series, no SSI was observed in the 70 recipients during the first 30 days after transplantation.

We observed 1 case of graft failure caused by hyperacute rejection on POD 8 and 2 deaths. One patient died of fulminant line sepsis, and the other death was a patient with a history of aortic dissection and aortoiliac stent placement; it was a complex case, which demanded complex vascular reconstruction at the backbench. According to the autopsy report, the patient died as a result of intra-abdominal hemorrhage on POD 6 at home.

We performed a case-control study in which the first 28 robotic-assisted kidney transplants were compared with a frequency-matched retrospective cohort of obese recipients who underwent kidney transplantation by open technique. We observed 1 wound complication in this robotic group, which was a hematoma in a patient on anticoagulation. No SSI was observed in this sample of robotic-assisted kidney transplanted obese recipients compared with 28% in the control group, and up to 40% in previous studies.[5] Based on the experience, we can state that robotic-assisted kidney transplantation for obese recipients is a safe and effective operation.

Current medical treatment of obesity often fails to achieve significant weight loss and long-term maintenance of lost weight. Thus, bariatric surgery is an effective modality to achieve significant long-term weight loss.[21] In order to attain the problem of obesity and its associated comorbidities in patients with ESRD, we proposed a prospective randomized trial designed to compare simultaneous robotic bariatric surgery and robotic LD kidney transplantation to robotic transplantation alone in obese patients with ESRD, approved by Institutional Review Board (protocol 2012-0014). The first patient included in the trial has had excellent outcomes. Her BMI decreased 10 points (from 42 kg/m^2 to 32 kg/m^2) at 6 months after transplant, preserving adequate graft function. Nevertheless, more patients and further results will elucidate whether the combined procedure is superior to renal transplantation alone in obese recipients.

By achieving adequate kidney graft function and minimizing surgical complications, robotic-assisted renal transplantation gives an opportunity to the disadvantaged group of obese patients with ESRD to have more realistic access to transplantation. However, robotic surgery in organ transplantation is an advance application of the technique, and a level of expertise is needed in any surgeon who considers this approach.

REFERENCES

1. Boggi U, Signori S, Vistoli F, et al. Laparoscopic robot-assisted pancreas transplantation: first world experience. Transplantation 2012;93(2):201–6.
2. Giulianotti PC, Tzvetanov I, Jeon H, et al. Robot-assisted right lobe donor hepatectomy. Transpl Int 2012;25(1):e5–9.
3. Friedman AN, Miskulin DC, Rosenberg IH, et al. Demographics and trends in overweight and obesity in patients at time of kidney transplantation. Am J Kidney Dis 2003;41(2):480–7.
4. Zaydfudim V, Feurer ID, Moore DR, et al. Pre-transplant overweight and obesity do not affect physical quality of life after kidney transplantation. J Am Coll Surg 2010;210(3):336–44.
5. Lynch RJ, Ranney DN, Shijie C, et al. Obesity, surgical site infection, and outcome following renal transplantation. Ann Surg 2009;250(6):1014–20.
6. Segev DL, Simpkins CE, Thompson RE, et al. Obesity impacts access to kidney transplantation. J Am Soc Nephrol 2008;19(2):349–55.
7. National Kidney Foundation. K/DOQI clinical practice guidelines for chronic kidney disease: evaluation, classification, and stratification. Am J Kidney Dis 2002; 39(2 Suppl 1):S1–266.
8. Scandling JD. Kidney transplant candidate evaluation. Semin Dial 2005;18(6): 487–94.
9. Vajdic CM, McDonald SP, McCredie MR, et al. Cancer incidence before and after kidney transplantation. JAMA 2006;296(23):2823–31.
10. Girndt M, Kohler H. Waiting time for patients with history of malignant disease before listing for organ transplantation. Transplantation 2005;80(Suppl 1): S167–70.
11. Bunnapradist S, Danovitch GM. Evaluation of adult kidney transplant candidates. Am J Kidney Dis 2007;50(5):890–8.
12. Kasiske BL, Cangro CB, Hariharan S, et al. The evaluation of renal transplantation candidates: clinical practice guidelines. Am J Transplant 2001;1(Suppl 2):3–95.
13. Gallon LG, Leventhal JR, Kaufman DB. Pretransplant evaluation of renal transplant candidates. Semin Nephrol 2002;22(6):515–25.

14. Kasiske BL, Klinger D. Cigarette smoking in renal transplant recipients. J Am Soc Nephrol 2000;11(4):753–9.
15. Gross CR, Kreitzer MJ, Russas V, et al. Mindfulness meditation to reduce symptoms after organ transplant: a pilot study. Adv Mind Body Med 2004;20(2):20–9.
16. Meier-Kriesche HU, Kaplan B. Waiting time on dialysis as the strongest modifiable risk factor for renal transplant outcomes: a paired donor kidney analysis. Transplantation 2002;74(10):1377–81.
17. Cupples CK, Cashion AK, Cowan PA, et al. Characterizing dietary intake and physical activity affecting weight gain in kidney transplant recipients. Prog Transplant 2012;22(1):62–70.
18. Phillips S, Heuberger R. Metabolic disorders following kidney transplantation. J Ren Nutr 2012;22(5):451–60.e451.
19. Giulianotti P, Gorodner V, Sbrana F, et al. Robotic transabdominal kidney transplantation in a morbidly obese patient. Am J Transplant 2010;10(6):1478–82.
20. Boggi U, Vistoli F, Signori S, et al. Robotic renal transplantation: first European case. Transpl Int 2011;24(2):213–8.
21. Tafti BA, Haghdoost M, Alvarez L, et al. Recovery of renal function in a dialysis-dependent patient following gastric bypass surgery. Obes Surg 2009;19(9):1335–9.

Left Lobe Liver Transplants

Lokesh Bathla, MD, Luciano M. Vargas, MD, Alan Langnas, DO*

KEYWORDS

- Adult • Left lobe liver transplantation • Living donor liver transplantation
- Small-for-size • Graft inflow modification

KEY POINTS

- Left lobe (LL) living-donor liver transplantation (LDLT) is safe and effective treatment for end-stage liver disease.
- LL LDLT shifts the risks of transplantation from the donor to the recipient, as the risk of donor morbidity and mortality are directly proportional to the extent of hepatectomy and the remnant liver volume.
- The risk of small-for-size syndrome in the recipient has prevented the use of LL allograft in the past. Various direct and indirect techniques for graft inflow modification (GIM) to control portal venous flow have essentially eliminated these risks.
- Two clinical forms of GIM include indirect reduction of portal flow by splenic artery ligation or splenectomy, and direct modulation of the portal flow by surgical construction of portosystemic shunts.
- LL LDLT, when performed with GIM where indicated, has long-term outcomes as good as those with cadaveric LT.
- Preference should be given to LL LDLT whenever possible, as this is safer for the donor and is also ethically correct.

INTRODUCTION

Living-donor liver transplantation (LDLT) is an established modality for the treatment of end-stage liver disease (ESLD). LDLT was first performed in children in 1989 using the left lateral segment (LLS) from an adult donor.[1] Encouraged by the success in children, LDLT was subsequently performed in adults in 1993 using a left lobe (LL) allograft.[2]

Although more than 5000 cadaveric liver transplants are performed annually in the United States, the rate of cadaveric liver transplantation has been stagnant for the last several years, with a wait-list mortality of nearly 25%.[3] Despite adoption of several strategies to combat this organ shortage, including use of split-liver transplantation, and donors who are older, hemodynamically unstable, have antibodies to hepatitis B or C virus, or donate after cardiac death (DCD), the expansion of the donor pool has been marginal. A strategy with great potential to address this problem of donor

Section of Transplant Surgery, University of Nebraska Medical Center, 983285 Nebraska Medical Center, Omaha, NE 68198-3285, USA
* Corresponding author.
E-mail address: alangnas@unmc.edu

Surg Clin N Am 93 (2013) 1325–1342
http://dx.doi.org/10.1016/j.suc.2013.09.003
0039-6109/13/$ – see front matter © 2013 Elsevier Inc. All rights reserved.
surgical.theclinics.com

shortage would be LDLT. Despite the vast potential for LDLT, concerns about donor safety continue to limit its expansion in Western countries.

The risk of donor morbidity and mortality are directly proportional to the extent of hepatectomy and the remnant liver volume in the donor, being least for LLS and highest for right lobe (RL) donation. From the recipient standpoint, adequacy of the graft volume (GV) is the most important determinant for a successful outcome, which should be at least 40% of the recipient's standard liver volume (SLV). Initially, LDLT was performed using the LL because of the familiarity of LLS LDLT in the pediatric population and the relatively lower morbidity with LL hepatectomy. In most of these instances, the GV was less than 40% of the recipient's SLV. Use of such allografts led to inferior outcomes in the recipients, in both the short- and long-term. In one of the early series, LL recipients in whom the graft-to-recipient weight ratio (GRWR) was less than 0.8, graft survival at 3 months was only 54.5%.[4] The transplantation of such small-for-size grafts (SFSGs) caused an imbalance between the rate of liver regeneration and an increased demand of liver function, causing severe graft dysfunction known as the small-for-size syndrome (SFSS). Dahm and colleagues[5] defined SFSS as GRWR less than 0.8% with 2 or more of the following findings on 3 consecutive days within the first week after transplantation: a bilirubin level greater than 10 mg/dL, an International Normalized Ratio (INR) greater than 2.0, and encephalopathy of grade 3 to 4. The etiology of SFSS is multifactorial, with portal hyperperfusion being the major causative factor.[6,7] Studies using animal models with partial liver transplants have reported sinusoidal congestion, rupture, and hemorrhage within minutes of reperfusion in the allograft. These changes, however, are not seen in full liver allografts, and their severity is inversely related to the size of allograft.[8] Additional findings from animal studies have also shown that these changes are reduced with partial diversion of the portal flow, and lead to improved graft function.[9,10] Based on these observations, the RL became the allograft of choice despite the relatively higher risk of morbidity and mortality to the donor.

Cumulative experience with LDLT over the last 2 decades, better understanding of the pathophysiology of SFSS, and the successful application of graft inflow modification (GIM) have made the issue of GV less important. Several centers have shown that small GV, defined as GV/SLV less than 40% and GRWR of 0.6%, in combination with GIM can be successfully used for LDLT with outcomes similar to those for cadaveric liver transplantation.[11,12]

In light of these technical refinements, the relatively lower risk of complications with LL LDLT with comparable outcomes, and the overriding concern for donor safety; it can be argued that LL allograft should be the graft of choice for LDLT whenever possible. Utilization of LL as the graft of choice fundamentally shifts the risks of LDLT from the donor to the recipient. In this article, the authors describe their operative technique of LL hepatectomy for LDLT and the use of various GIM techniques. Patient selection, perioperative management, and donor outcomes as relevant are also discussed.

PREOPERATIVE PLANNING

The evaluation of a potential donor for LDLT is a 3-step process that involves (1) clinical assessment and serologic testing, (2) radiologic imaging, and (3) liver biopsy (optional).

Any healthy adult between the age of 18 and 60 years who is ABO compatible can be a donor for LDLT. A complete history and physical examination is performed, including body weight and height measurement to calculate the body mass index (BMI). Laboratory testing includes complete blood count, serum chemistries, thyroid function tests, coagulation profile, and screening for hepatitis A, B, and C, human immunodeficiency virus, Epstein-Barr virus, cytomegalovirus, syphilis, hypercholesterolemia, common causes of hypercoagulability, and diabetes mellitus. Mammography, colonoscopy, Papanicolaou smear, and prostate-specific antigen results must be up to date according to current health-maintenance guidelines.[13] Antimitochondrial antibody screen should be performed in donors with a family history of primary biliary cirrhosis. The donor should also be seen by a mental health care professional for psychological/psychiatric evaluation. The donor should not have any active or uncontrolled psychiatric disorder. There should be no psychosocial, motivational, or ethical issues with the donor. Donors who smoke must abstain for at least 6 weeks before the surgery. In the case of female donors, oral contraceptives are stopped once donor evaluation is initiated. The authors also obtain cardiac clearance in donors with comorbidities such as hypertension or if they are older than 50 years.

Individuals who are deemed to be suitable candidates on clinical and serologic assessment undergo radiologic assessment to delineate the anatomy of the liver, the hepatic veins, portal vein, hepatic artery, and biliary system; volumetric analysis of individual lobes; and assessment of the degree of hepatic steatosis. Magnetic resonance imaging (MRI) with magnetic resonance cholangiopancreatography (MRCP) is the authors' investigation modality of choice, although institutional practices may vary. The spatial resolution of MRCP for defining the intrahepatic biliary anatomy is often inadequate, especially when the donor biliary tree is inherently small in caliber or there is excessive patient movement during testing.[14]

Accurate size matching of the donor and recipient is essential to ensure that adequate functional hepatic mass is available to the recipient to sustain metabolic needs, permit regeneration, and avoid SFSS. Volumetric assessment of the RL and LL are performed to ascertain the side and extent of hepatectomy needed. From the recipient standpoint, an estimated GRWR of 0.8% is required. Graft weight to SLV of recipient should be about 30% to 40%. Concurrently, the remnant liver volume should be at least 30% to 40% of the original liver volume in the donor, assuming that the residual liver parenchyma is normal. Specialized software such as the MeVis Liver Analyzer and Liver View (MeVis Medical Imaging, Bremen, Germany) assists in this decision-making process by producing 3-dimensional liver models for volume measurements (**Fig. 1**), preoperative planning of surgical planes, and identifying vascular and biliary variations that can affect the allograft size or contraindicate hepatectomy altogether. Several studies on imaging-based volumetric techniques have been published showing good correlation between the actual GVs and radiologically assessed graft volume, with a margin of error ranging from 5% to 25%.[15,16] The main cause of these discrepancies is related to graft perfusion, because imaging measures the volume of the perfused liver, whereas weight measurements of the actual graft are performed when it is devoid of blood.

The comprehensive road map provided by the imaging not only facilitates detailed surgical planning but also reduces postoperative complications in the donor and the recipient. Variations in hepatic arterial anatomy are encountered in nearly 45% of cases (**Fig. 2**).[17] Presence of a variant dominant supply to segment IV by the right hepatic artery (in nearly 11% of cases) is a significant anomaly for LL transplants, as double arterial anastomoses (left hepatic artery [LHA] and segment IV variant artery) may be necessary. Identification of separate origins of the segment II and III branches from the proper hepatic artery are also important, as this may also require multiple arterial anastomoses. Variations in hepatic venous and portal venous anatomy are not as common for LL allografts, making an LL allograft technically easier to harvest and implant (**Fig. 3**).

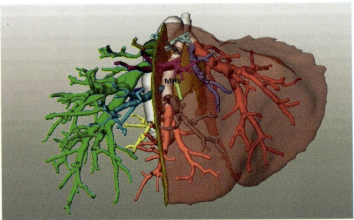

Cut1, Left Lobe Graft with MHV (Volumes)

	Territory	Volume	Relative (%)
	Cutting Plane	18 ml	1.2
	Graft	625 ml	44.2
	Remnant	771 ml	54.5
	Total	1414 ml	100.0

Fig. 1. MeVis reconstruction showing left lobe allograft with portal venous and hepatic venous territories. Estimated graft and remnant volumes based on the volumetric analysis are also shown. MHV, middle hepatic vein.

Variations in biliary anatomy are present in nearly 40% of the population (**Fig. 4**). Detailed study of the biliary anatomy is critical for LDLT, as biliary complications are the most common complications in both donors and recipients. Significant biliary variants include common hepatic duct trifurcation, drainage of the right hepatic duct system in the left duct system, and drainage of the right posterior duct into the left main duct.

The role of preoperative donor liver biopsy is controversial, and practices vary around the world. According to the Vancouver Forum guidelines, a donor liver biopsy should be performed in cases of abnormal liver function tests and evidence of

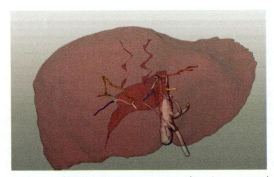

Fig. 2. MeVis reconstruction of hepatic artery anatomy showing a completely replaced right and left hepatic artery.

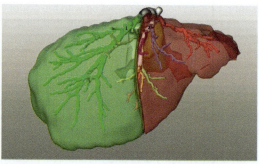

Fig. 3. MeVis reconstruction of liver, showing 3-dimensional reconstruction of hepatic veins and division of the right and left lobe along the principal plane immediately to the right of middle hepatic vein. 1, right hepatic vein; 2, middle hepatic vein; 3, left hepatic vein.

steatosis, or if other abnormalities are noted on imaging studies.[18] In addition, preoperative liver biopsy should be considered in donors genetically related to recipients with autoimmune hepatitis, primary sclerosing cholangitis, or primary biliary cirrhosis, or donors with a BMI greater than 30 kg/m^2.[18] Because this is an invasive part of the donor evaluation and can have its own complications, it is usually performed just before scheduling the LDLT so that one is able to rule out other exclusion criteria.

CONSENT

Voluntary and informed consent can be summarized as the primary selection criterion for LDLT donation. The donor should understand the possibility of primary nonfunction, recurrence of liver disease in the allograft, graft loss attributable to technical reasons, or rejection and death of the recipient. At our center, we provide the LDLT donor candidates with information about our experience with LDLT, cadaveric LT, complex hepatobiliary surgeries, and short- and long-term donor morbidities, mortality, and donor

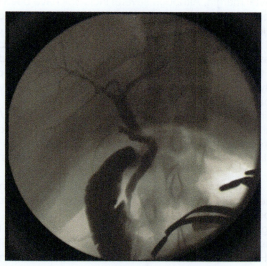

Fig. 4. Intraoperative cholangiogram showing biliary hilar trifurcation in a left lobe donor.

outcomes. The consent process should be reviewed with the donor in private to ensure there is no coercion. The donor should be made aware that he or she has the right to withdraw from the process at any time until the time of surgery.

ANESTHESIA MANAGEMENT

The goal of anesthesia management is to provide the safest anesthetic with minimal morbidity, and address issues such as hypothermia, maintenance of low central venous pressure (CVP), and postoperative analgesia. The anesthesia-related risks to a live liver donor are no more than those of general anesthesia for any complex abdominal surgery.

The authors use both chemoprophylaxis and mechanical prophylaxis against deep venous thrombosis (DVT) in all donors. During the hepatectomy phase of the operation, the CVP is maintained at low levels (0–5 cm) with a combination of fluid restriction and venodilatory agents if necessary. Because sympathetic stimulation during anesthesia induction can raise the CVP, measures such as reduction of preoperative anxiety with the use of anxiolytics, minimizing sympathetic stimulation during intubation and maintenance of adequate depth of anesthesia are important. The authors do not use homologous or autologous blood transfusions for the donors. Storage of autologous blood is used by several centers in the setting of right liver donation.[18] The authors use a cell-saver device to minimize the blood loss in all cases.

An arterial line and 9F central venous catheter are placed for invasive monitoring and rapid fluid administration if necessary. Attention is paid to avoid hypothermia in the donor by monitoring room temperature as well as active warming of the patient with hot-air devices. Placement of a nasogastric tube and Foley catheter is performed in all patients. The patient is placed in the supine position with the right arm extended at 90° and left arm placed at the side. Appropriate antibiotic prophylaxis is administered within 60 minutes before the incision as per the institutional protocol.

DONOR HEPATECTOMY

- A right subcostal incision with left subcostal extension is made 2 finger breadths below the costal margin. Although several incisions have been described for left donor hepatectomy, this incision is preferred for the ease of mobilization of both right and left lobes and access to the retrohepatic inferior vena cava (IVC). Occasionally, a midline extension toward the xiphoid process may be required in patients who have a deep abdominal cavity extending high up under the rib cage to gain access to the insertion of the hepatic veins. Laparoscopic-assisted and, more recently, completely laparoscopic hepatectomies for live donation have been described, but are not currently standard of care.
- Bimanual palpation of the liver is performed to estimate the GV, as preoperative estimates can occasionally be misleading (see above). The falciform ligament is taken down to its insertion at the junction of the hepatic veins and the IVC.
- A self-retaining retractor system is then set up to establish the necessary exposure.
- At this point intraoperative ultrasonography (IOUS) is performed to review the portal and hepatic venous anatomy, and evaluate for any occult lesions that might have been missed on preoperative imaging.
- The left triangular ligament is then divided to mobilize the LLS. Dissection is carried out all the way to the level of insertion of the left phrenic vein into the left hepatic vein (LHV). This dissection is carried medially until the medial aspects of both the LHV the IVC are exposed.

- The confluence of the LHV and the middle hepatic vein (MHV) is then exposed. Low insertions of the left phrenic vein and ligamentum venosum are divided to expose the medial aspect of the LHV. Occasionally, the LHV inserts low into the IVC and the confluence is covered with hepatic parenchyma from the caudate lobe. In these situations, the overlying liver tissue is divided to expose the junction of the LHV and IVC.
- The hepatoduodenal and hepatogastric ligaments are exposed by retracting the LLS cephalad and distal stomach caudally. The hepatogastric ligament is then divided. Accessory or replaced LHA, if present, is encountered in this ligament and is preserved. These aberrant vessels are then carefully dissected all the way to their origin from the left gastric artery.
- The hepatoduodenal ligament is opened along its most medial aspect to expose the LHA. The LHA is dissected proximally up to its origin from the hepatic artery proper. Distally the LHA is dissected until the anterior surface of the left portal vein (LPV) is exposed. Dissection the proper hepatic artery is not necessary and is discouraged, as this may injure the arterial blood supply to the remnant liver.
- The LHA is gently retracted with a vessel loop laterally to allow for anterior exposure of the LPV. The LPV is then mobilized circumferentially. Often short portal branches to segment IV are encountered, which are divided between fine silk ligatures.
- The tissue along the medial aspect of the hilar plate is divided to allow for additional retraction of the quadrate lobe cephalad. This action helps with the identification of the left hepatic duct cephalad to the LHA and anterior to the LPV.
- The confluence of the right and left hepatic ducts is dissected out. Care should be taken not to skeletonize the ducts during this dissection, as it may compromise its blood supply and cause biliary complications.
- A large hemoclip is placed on the periductal tissue at the anticipated site of transection (**Fig. 5**). The gallbladder is mobilized using the fundus-first approach. A transcystic cholangiogram is then performed to confirm the biliary anatomy, identify any occult accessory ducts not identified on preoperative imaging, and determine the location of the hepatic duct confluence in relation to the hemoclip.

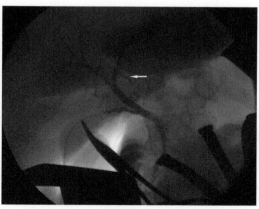

Fig. 5. Intraoperative cholangiogram demonstrating the biliary ductal anatomy and the hemoclip (*arrow*) confirming the proposed site of left hepatic duct transection.

- The caudate lobe is mobilized by dividing the peritoneum along its left border extending from the level of hepatic veins superiorly to its inferior border, where it is attached to the IVC. When freeing the caudate lobe from the IVC, several small direct hepatic venous branches from the caudate lobe to the IVC are encountered. These branches can be either ligated with fine silk ties or divided using a tissue-sealing device such as LigaSure Precise (Valleylab Inc, Boulder, CO, USA).
- IOUS is performed again to identify the course of the hepatic veins as well as any hepatic vein branches traversing the plane of transection. The liver capsule is then marked with diathermy 1 cm to the right of the course of the MHV; this marks the anterior projection of the plane of parenchymal transection, and extends posteriorly to the anterior surface of the IVC.
- At this point the left hepatic duct is sharply transected at the level that was determined by the intraoperative cholangiogram.
- A Penrose drain is passed posterior to the liver, in front of the hilar structures inferiorly. It is brought out superiorly anterior to the IVC and to the right of the MHV.
- Parenchymal transection is initiated in the gallbladder fossa. The dissection is then continued with the Cavitron Ultrasonic Surgical Aspirator (CUSA system 200; Valleylab Inc, Boulder, Colorado, USA).
- When the recipient team is ready and parenchymal transection has been completed, the patient is anticoagulated with 60 U/kg heparin intravenously (**Fig. 6**). The LHA is ligated and divided sharply. A vascular clamp is then placed on the LPV, which is then divided sharply. The MHV and LHV are then clamped distal to their confluence close to the IVC and divided sharply.
- The specimen is transferred to the back table and flushed with cold preservative solution, and transferred to the recipient room on ice.
- The stumps of the hepatic vein and portal vein are oversewn with nonabsorbable polypropylene suture. The stump of the left hepatic duct is oversewn with 6-0 Maxon or PDS suture in a running fashion.
- The cut surface of the liver is then examined for any evidence of bleeding and bile leakage. Small ducts transected during the parenchymal dissection are identified and oversewn with 6-0 Maxon suture.
- A closed-suction drain is placed along the cut surface of the liver. The abdomen is closed in a standard 2-layer fashion with heavy absorbable sutures.

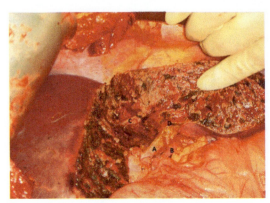

Fig. 6. Completed left lobe parenchymal transection showing left portal vein (A), left hepatic artery (B), middle hepatic vein (C), and left hepatic duct (D).

- The patient is then extubated in the operating room and transferred to the post-anesthesia care unit (PACU), and subsequently transferred to the intensive care unit (ICU) for the first 24 hours.

RECIPIENT HEPATECTOMY AND IMPLANTATION

- A standard right subcostal incision with left extension is made to enter the abdominal cavity, followed by mobilization of the liver in a fashion akin to that of cadaveric transplantation.
- After mobilization of both the right and left lobe, hilar dissection is performed. The right hepatic artery and LHA are individually ligated. The common bile duct is divided as high as possible. Right, left, and main portal veins are circumferentially dissected.
- Liver is then mobilized off the retrohepatic IVC followed by isolation of the right, middle, and left hepatic veins.
- Clamps are placed across the main portal vein and the hepatic veins proximal to their insertion in the IVC.
- Right and left portal veins are then divided, followed by division of the right, middle, and left hepatic veins close to the liver.
- At this point, a decision is made regarding creation of a hemi-portacaval shunt (HPCS), depending on the weight of the allograft. If the GW/RW ratio is less than 0.8, the authors routinely perform splenic artery ligation. The decision to perform HPCS is made if portal venous pressure is greater than 15 mm Hg or if portal venous flow (PVF) to the allograft will be greater than 250 mL/min/100 g liver tissue. At times simple venting of the native portal vein can provide some idea of portal vein flow.
- The right portal vein is anastomosed to the IVC in an end-to-side fashion to create the HPCS. A large hemoclip is applied on the anterior surface of IVC adjacent to the shunt. This clip acts as a radiopaque marker to locate the site of HPCS during endovascular closure of the shunt, if needed.
- The orifice of the right hepatic vein is oversewn. The intervening septum between the MHV and LHV is divided to create single common orifice.
- Allograft is introduced to the field, and the common orifice of the donor hepatic veins is anastomosed to the common orifice of the recipient's hepatic veins using 4-0 polypropylene suture.
- The donor LPV is anastomosed to the recipient LPV in a running fashion using 6-0 polypropylene suture.
- The LHA of the donor is anastomosed to the recipient's left or common hepatic artery, depending on the best size match between the donor and recipient.
- Clamps are released at this point, and the allograft is reperfused (**Fig. 7**). Bleeding points (if any) at anastomotic sites or cut surface of liver are controlled. Using a flow meter, blood flow is measured in the right portal vein, LPV, and middle portal vein (MPV). Alternatively, direct pressure measurements are performed in the MPV. If the pressure in the MPV is greater than 15 mm or the MPV flow is greater than 250 mL/min/100 g liver tissue after unclamping, GIM is indicated and the HPCS is left open.
- Patients in whom the portal flow to the allograft is less than 250 mL/min/100 g liver tissue, test occlusion of the HPCS is performed and the flow to the allograft is reevaluated. For patients who tolerate the test occlusion without an increase in the portal flow to more than 250 mL/min/100 g liver tissue, the shunt is ligated to prevent portal steal.

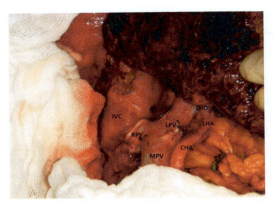

Fig. 7. Left lobe allograft with hemi-portacaval shunt and complete vascularization. CHA, common hepatic artery; IVC, inferior vena cava; LHA, donor left hepatic artery; LHD, left hepatic duct; LPV, left portal vein; MPV, main portal vein; RPV, right portal vein.

- Biliary-enteric continuity is established by performing either a Roux-en-Y hepaticojejunostomy or duct-to-duct biliary anastomosis.
- A closed suction drain is placed along the cut surface of the liver. The allograft is oriented in its anatomic position by suspending to the falciform ligament to prevent torsion.
- The abdomen is closed in 2 layers and the patient is transferred to the ICU in intubated condition.

POSTOPERATIVE MANAGEMENT (DONOR)

After observation in the ICU for the first 24 hours, the patients are transferred to the surgical floor. The nasogastric tube and urinary catheter are removed. Patients are started on a clear liquid diet if tolerated. Pain is controlled with intravenous narcotics using patient-controlled analgesia (PCA), and they are also started on chemoprophylaxis against DVT on the morning after surgery. Aggressive pulmonary toilet using incentive spirometer and early ambulation with assistance is strongly encouraged. Routine laboratory tests are done for the first 48 to 72 hours to monitor for hemoglobin and liver functions. Drains are removed on postoperative day 2 or 3, provided the output is not bilious and patient is tolerating diet. Patients are usually discharged on postoperative day 4 or 5, provided they are ambulatory, tolerating diet, and their pain is well controlled with oral medications.

POSTOPERATIVE MANAGEMENT (RECIPIENT)

Patients are transferred to the ICU in intubated condition. Sedation and paralytic agents are withheld, allowing the patients to breathe spontaneously and wake up. Once the patients are awake and alert, they are extubated. Ultrasonography of the allograft is performed to ensure patency of the vessels of the allograft. Serum chemistries, blood counts, coagulation profile, and blood gases are monitored every 6 hours for the first 24 hours and subsequently on a daily basis. The INR is usually elevated in the first 48 to 72 hours postoperatively as the allograft regenerates. The authors usually do not correct elevated INR unless there is evidence of bleeding or the INR is higher than 3.5. Hypophosphatemia is common and should be aggressively corrected. Cholestasis is common in the early postoperative period, especially when GRWR is less than 0.8. Elevation in serum creatinine is not uncommon during the first week postoperatively, mostly as a result of intravascular dehydration, calcineurin inhibitor toxicity, or rarely due to sepsis. Careful attention is paid to the volume status, as there is a tendency for fluid retention with SFSG, and the patient may be intravascularly dry despite overall positive fluid balance. Patients usually spend 24 to 48 hours in the ICU and are then transferred to the surgical floor. Clinical assessment to rule out encephalopathy is performed on a daily basis, as it may be a sign of "portal steal phenomenon." Any deviation in the patient's postoperative clinical course should prompt thorough workup. The first step is to perform ultrasonography of the allograft to ensure patency of vasculature and rule out complex fluid collections. Sepsis workup is initiated if the patient has fever, hypotension, and/or alteration in mental status. Patients who have elevations in liver function tests undergo liver biopsy to rule out rejection. In patients who show signs of encephalopathy, HPCS should be closed either by open means or endovascularly.[19] Immunosuppression for these patients consists of steroids and tacrolimus. The target level of tacrolimus for the first month is between 10 and 15 ng/mL. Clear liquid diet is started on postoperative day 1, and advanced as tolerated. Drains are removed once the patient is tolerating diet and the output is nonbilious. Patients are usually discharged on postoperative day 7 or 8.

COMPLICATIONS (DONOR)

A wide variety of complications ranging from perineal nerve palsy to death have been reported in the literature in patients undergoing live liver donor surgery. In addition, the incidence of such complications as reported in the literature varies widely, because a uniform definition as to what constitutes a complication is lacking. The Vancouver Forum recommended use of the Clavien system to record and grade live donor complications by severity (**Box 1**).[18] A list of all complications in the recently reported Adult-to-Adult Live Donor Liver Transplant (A2ALL) cohort study is provided in **Box 2**.[18]

COMPLICATIONS (RECIPIENT)

Complications in the recipients of LL LDLT include vascular complications, biliary complications, sepsis, massive ascites, SFSS, portal steal phenomenon, and rejection. There is a lack of well-defined data about vascular complications in the published literature in patients undergoing LDLT. It would be reasonable to assume that incidence of vascular complications in LDLT would be at least as frequent as seen with cadaveric transplantation. Depending on how soon hepatic artery thrombosis or portal vein thrombosis is identified, graft salvage can be attempted. Unfortunately, this is not always successful, and the patient is listed for retransplantation.

Biliary complications associated with LDLT include bile leak, stricture, and cholangitis. If detected early enough, these complications warrant operative repair. Often, these leaks are managed successfully with conservative management. Some of them heal with stricture formation and eventually require operative repair. Episodes of cholangitis are treated with antibiotics, and biliary imaging is performed to rule out biliary stricture as the cause of cholangitis. These strictures can be managed with either balloon dilation or operative repair (mostly the latter).

Patients undergoing LDLT with an allograft whereby the GRWR is less than 0.8 usually undergo HPCS to prevent graft dysfunction in the early postoperative period, as mentioned earlier. Not infrequently, these patients develop portal steal phenomenon whereby, owing to the low resistance in the HPCS, the portal flow from the liver is diverted to the shunt. These patients present with encephalopathy, elevated bilirubin,

> **Box 1**
> **Clavien classification of surgical complications adapted for live liver donors: grades**
>
> - Grade 1: Non–life-threatening complications
>
>   Require interventions only at the bedside
>
>   Postoperative bleeding of less than 4 units of packed red blood cells
>
>   Never associated with prolongation of intensive care unit (ICU) or hospital stay longer than twice the median of the population in study
>
> - Grade 2: No residual disability
>
>   2a: Require only use of medication or 4 or more units of packed red blood cells
>
>   2b: Require therapeutic interventions, readmission to the hospital or ICU, or prolongation of regular ICU stay for more than 5 days
>
>   2c: Any potential donor who has an aborted surgery. Donor surgery does not result in transplantation
>
> - Grade 3: Residual disability
>
>   3a: There is low risk of death that results in permanent but not progressive disability
>
>   3b: There is lasting disability that is either difficult to control or has a significant risk of death or liver failure
>
> - Grade 4: Liver failure or death
>
>   4a: Lead to liver transplantation
>
>   4b: Lead to donor death
>
> *Data from* Barr ML, Belghiti J, Villamil FG, et al. A report of the Vancouver Forum on the care of the live organ donor: lung, liver, pancreas, and intestine data and medical guidelines. Transplantation 2006;81:1373–85.

and, occasionally, elevated liver enzymes. Ultrasonographic examination of the allograft reveals patent vasculature, thereby ruling out vascular cause for the patient's clinical state. Closure of the shunt is indicated in these patients, and can be performed by the open or endovascular technique as mentioned earlier.

DISCUSSION

In the current era, LDLT has become increasingly safe from the donor standpoint, and has long-term outcomes as good as those for cadaveric liver transplants. Although more than 11,000 LDLTs have been performed worldwide, the issue of donor safety continues to be of prime importance, and rightfully so. A total of 34 living liver donor deaths have been reported in the literature of the 11,553 donor hepatectomies so far, mostly with RL donation.[13] Episodes of living liver donor mortality were especially emphasized in the United States fairly recently, raising serious concerns about donor safety. There is a significant difference in the incidence of morbidity and mortality when RL donation is compared with LL donation. Hwang and colleagues[20] reported their experience of more than 1000 LDLTs with an overall major donor complication (Clavien grade III and higher) rate of 3.2% and no mortality. The major donor complication rate was 4.9% (29 of 591) for RL donors and 1.4% (8 of 571) for LL donors in this study. Taketomi and colleagues[21] reported their cumulative experience of 206 LDLT with an overall complication rate of 34%. These investigators observed a significantly higher complication rate in RL donors when compared with LL donors

---

Box 2
Complications recorded in the Adult-to-Adult Live Donor Liver Transplant (A2ALL) study

- Intraoperative injury
  - Bile duct
  - Hepatic artery
  - Portal vein
- Biliary complications
  - Bile leak/biloma
  - Biliary stricture
- Abdominal/Gastrointestinal
  - Intra-abdominal bleeding
  - Gastrointestinal bleeding
  - Localized intra-abdominal abscess
  - Ileus (delayed return of bowel function for >7 days)
  - Bowel obstruction
  - Reexploration
- Cardiopulmonary
  - Myocardial infarction
  - Congestive heart failure
  - Pneumothorax (requiring chest tube)
  - Pleural effusion (requiring thoracentesis)
  - Pulmonary edema
  - Cardiopulmonary arrest
  - Respiratory arrest
  - Aspiration
  - Pulmonary embolism
- Wound complications
  - Dehiscence
  - Hernia development
- Liver-specific events
  - Encephalopathy
  - Ascites
  - Liver failure
  - Hepatic artery thrombosis
  - Portal vein thrombosis
  - Inferior vena cava thrombosis
  - Transplantation
- General
  - Deep venous thrombosis
  - Neuropraxia

○ Infections

○ Psychological: depression, suicide, other

Data from Barr ML, Belghiti J, Villamil FG, et al. A report of the Vancouver Forum on the care of the live organ donor: lung, liver, pancreas, and intestine data and medical guidelines. Transplantation 2006;81:1373–85.

(43.4% vs 29.2%, *P*<.05). Biliary complication rates in their study were 2.9% for LL and 10.1% for RL (*P*<.05). There was no significant difference in graft survival up to 5 years after transplantation. In another review of more than 1600 living donor hepatectomies, the morbidity rates were 8.2% for 753 LLS donors, 12% for 484 LL donors, and 19% for 443 RL donors.[22] In addition, the biliary fistula rate in this study was 10% in RL donors and 2% in LL donors. In another large retrospective analysis of more than 1200 living liver donors from a single center, Iida and colleagues[23] observed a significantly higher rate of major complications (Clavien grade IIIa–V) with RL and extended RL grafts compared with non-RL grafts (44.2% vs 18.8%, *P*<.05), and also reported 1 donor death attributed to hepatic failure after extended RL donation. Several other studies have shown similar results, with higher morbidity associated with RL donation in comparison with LL donation.[24,25] The most comprehensive review from the North American experience was reported in the Adult-to-Adult Living Donor Liver Transplant Cohort Study, which reported a near 40% complication rate with LDLT donor surgery. The study did not segregate complications of RL versus LL living liver donation. Of the 760 patients, only 33 were LL and 20 donor operations were aborted. There was no mortality reported in the study.[26]

From the recipient standpoint, concerns about SFSS have prevented the use of LL allograft in most instances. Various direct and indirect techniques for GIM have essentially eliminated the issue of SFSS. Patients in whom the GRWR is less than 0.8% are at risk of SFSS and should undergo GIM. GIM currently targets a portal venous pressure less than 15 to 20 mm Hg or PVF less than 250 mL/min/100 g of liver tissue. Two clinical forms of GIM include indirect reduction of portal flow by splenic artery ligation or splenectomy, and direct modulation of the portal flow by surgical construction of portosystemic shunts. There is no defined algorithm regarding which approach to use first. Splenic artery ligation can be tried first, as it is least invasive. For patients in whom PVF is >500 mL/min/100 g liver tissue, HPCS should be considered, as splenic artery ligation alone will not be effective. Troisi and colleagues,[27] who first described the technique of HPCS, reported a 1-year graft survival of 75% with the use of HPCS and 20% without HPCS in patients who underwent LDLT with GRWR of less than 0.8. The reduction in PVF by HPCS can sometimes be too much and may lead to the portal steal phenomenon: this risks hepatofugal flow, portal venous thrombosis, graft dysfunction, and encephalopathy. In these circumstances the HPCS needs to be taken down, either surgically or endovascularly, by placement of a covered stent in the infrahepatic IVC.[19] Several studies have shown that with the use of GIM, the GRWR can be safely reduced to 0.6%.[12,27–31] Botha and colleagues[30] reported their experience with 21 LL LDLT with a median GRWR of 0.67 (range 0.5–1.0), with HPCS performed in 16 patients. These investigators observed a reduction in the hepatic venous pressure gradient (HVPG) from a median of 18 to 5 mm Hg. Patient and graft survival in their cohort was 87% and 81%, respectively, at 12 months.

An alternative to HPCS that is being used more frequently is to perform splenectomy in patients with an HVPG greater than 14 mm Hg. Ikegami and colleagues[32] recently reported their experience of 250 LDLTs using LL grafts. Patients were divided into Era 1 (n = 121, where the surgical techniques were refined) and Era 2 (n = 129, where the established procedures were used). In Era 2, the GRWR was 0.71 ± 0.13, which was significantly lower than in Era1 (0.84 ± 0.25%, P<.01). In addition, the investigators observed significantly improved PVF in Era 2. Splenectomy was performed predominantly in Era 2 for GIM (7% vs 69%, P<.01). Ikegami and colleagues advocate splenectomy and ligation of major shunt vessels (>10 mm) to optimize portal dynamics. Another advantage of splenectomy is the reduction in hepatic vascular tonus with improved vascular compliance secondary to blockage of the endothelin-1 pathway, the spleen being the major source of endothelin-1 in the portal system. In summary, the use of GIM with LL grafts when GRWR is lower than 0.8% reduces the incidence of SFSS significantly. It also addresses the overriding concerns of donor safety by allowing the use of LL grafts, thereby reducing the morbidity and mortality of living liver donation. The use of LL grafts, despite GIM, should be limited to patients whose MELD (Model for End-Stage Liver Disease) score is 24 or less.

Kawasaki and colleagues[33] were the first to report short-term results with LL LDLT. These investigators performed LDLT using LL in 13 patients with a GV/SLV ratio ranging from 32% to 59%. Two patients in their cohort died 2.5 and 22 months after LDLT. The remaining 11 patients were doing well 2 to 35 months after transplantation. None of the patients in this group developed SFSS. In another study comprising 45 patients, Shimada and colleagues[34] reported on a comparison between right and left lobe grafts. Thirty-nine patients underwent LL donation, of which 24 included the caudate lobe. At 18 months after transplantation, the survival rate for RL grafts was 75% and that for LL grafts was 85.6%.

Soejima and colleagues[35] reported long-term outcomes on 200 consecutive LL LDLTs, which were compared retrospectively with 112 RL LDLTs. The mean GV/SLV ratio and GRWR were 38.7% (range 21.0%–66.1%) and 0.82% (range 0.41%–1.51%), respectively in LL grafts. These values were significantly smaller than those of RL grafts (47.4% and 0.9%, respectively). The cumulative overall 1-, 5-, and 10-year patient survival rates were 85.6%, 77.9%, and 69.5%, respectively, in LL LDLT. These rates were comparable with those of RL LDLT (89.8%, 71.3%, and 70.7%, respectively). Soejima and colleagues proposed an algorithm to help select the appropriate graft for LDLT (**Fig. 8**), recommending the use of LL as the graft of choice when possible. Several other studies have shown similar results, with excellent 1- and 5-year outcomes.[30,32,36–38]

The literature on LL adult-to-adult LDLT from North America is scant. Saidi and colleagues[39] analyzed retrospectively the data on LDLT reported between 1998 and 2010 to the United Network for Organ Sharing (UNOS) to study the impact of allograft selection of LL versus RL on outcome in recipients. Of 2844 patients who underwent LDLT, 2690 (94.6%) underwent RL LDLT and only 154 (5.4%) underwent LL LDLT. In Cox regression analysis, LL LDLT was associated with increased risk of graft failure (hazard ratio 2.39) and patient death (hazard ratio 1.86). The study concluded that LL LDLT was not ready for wider use based on recipient outcomes, although it was clearly a safer operation for the donor. This study failed to take into consideration other important determinants of success such as GRWR, SFSS, center and surgeon volume and experience, surgical techniques, and graft weight. The study failed to explain the increasing number of LL LDLT being performed in the United States, where LL LDLT represented only 2.3% of all LDLTs during 1998 to 2003, and 7.2% of all LDLTs in 2004 to 2010 (P = .01). Clearly the United States experience with LL LDLT is very limited in comparison with what has been reported in the worldwide literature. This trend, however, is changing with improved understanding of SFSS, techniques of

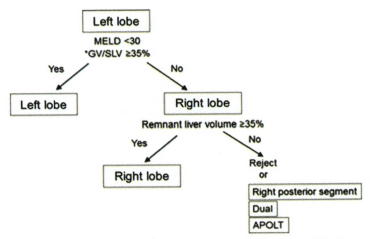

Fig. 8. Proposed algorithm for graft selection for LDLT. APOLT, auxiliary partial orthotopic liver transplantation; GV, graft volume; MELD, Model for End-Stage Liver Disease; SLV, standard liver volume. (*From* Soejima Y, Shirabe K, Taketomi A, et al. Left lobe living donor live transplantation in adults. Am J Transpl 2012;12:1879; with permission.)

GIM, and increasing frequency of LL LDLT. Botha and colleagues[30] reported the largest series of LL LDLT from North America, presenting data on 21 patients who underwent small-for-size LL LDLT with a mean GRWR of 0.67 (range 0.5–1.0). All of the patients in this series underwent HPCS for GIM. SFSS developed in only 1 patient, with 1-year patient and graft survival of 87% and 81%, respectively.

SUMMARY

LL LDLT is a safe and effective treatment for ESLD. From the donor standpoint, LL donation is clearly safer than RL donation. Although it transfers the risks of LDLT onto the recipient, various forms of GIM can mitigate such risks. There is ample evidence in the literature that LL LDLT, when performed with GIM where indicated, has long-term outcomes as good as those seen with cadaveric LT. Preference should be given to LL LDLT whenever possible, as this is safer for the donor and is also ethically right thing to do.

REFERENCES

1. Raia S, Nery JR, Mies S. Liver transplantation from live donors. Lancet 1989;2:497.
2. Hashikura Y, Makuuchi M, Kawasaki S, et al. Successful living related partial liver transplantation to an adult patient. Lancet 1994;343:1233–4.
3. Organ Procurement and Transplantation Network (OPTN) and Scientific Registry of Transplant Recipients (SRTR). OPTN/SRTR 2011 annual data report. Rockville (MD): Department of Health and Human Services, Health Resources and Services Administration, Healthcare Bureau, Division of Transplantation; 2012. p. 78–100.
4. Tanaka K, Ogura Y. "Small-for-size graft" and "small-for-size syndrome" in living donor liver transplantation. Yonsei Med J 2004;45:1089–94.

5. Dahm F, Georgiev P, Clavien PA. Small-for-size syndrome after partial liver transplantation: definition, mechanisms of disease and clinical implications. Am J Transplant 2005;5:2605–10.
6. Ito T, Kiuchi T, Yamamoto H, et al. Changes in portal venous pressure in the early phase after living donor living transplantation: pathogenesis and clinical implications. Transplantation 2003;75:1313–7.
7. Man K, Lo CM, Ng IO, et al. Liver transplantation in rats using small-for-size grafts: a study of hemodynamic and morphological changes. Arch Surg 2001; 136:280–5.
8. Kelly DM, Demetris AJ, Fung JJ, et al. Porcine partial liver transplantation: a novel model of the "small-for-size" liver graft. Liver Transpl 2004;10:253–63.
9. Boillot O, Delafosse B, Mècher I, et al. Small-for-size partial liver graft in an adult recipient; new transplant technique. Lancet 2002;359:406–7.
10. Wang HS, Ohkohchi N, Enomoto Y, et al. Excessive portal flow causes graft failure in extremely small-for-size liver transplantation in pigs. World J Gastroenterol 2005;11:6954–9.
11. Chan SC, Lo CM, Ng KK, et al. Alleviating the burden of small-for-size graft in right liver living donor liver transplantation through accumulation of experience. Am J Transplant 2010;10:859–67.
12. Kaido T, Mori A, Ogura Y, et al. Lower limit of the graft-to-recipient weight ratio can be safely reduced to 0.6% in adult-to-adult living donor liver transplantation in combination with portal pressure control. Transplant Proc 2011;43: 2391–3.
13. Roll GR, Parekh JR, Parker WF, et al. Left hepatectomy versus right hepatectomy for living donor liver transplantation: shifting the risk from the donor to the recipient. Liver Transpl 2013;19:472–81.
14. Fulcher AS, Szucs RA, Bassignani MJ, et al. Right lobe living donor liver transplantation: preoperative evaluation of the donor with MR imaging. AJR Am J Roentgenol 2001;176:1483–91.
15. Schiano TD, Bodian C, Schwartz ME, et al. Accuracy and significance of computed tomographic scan assessment of hepatic volume in patients undergoing liver transplantation. Transplantation 2000;69:545–50.
16. Harada N, Shimada M, Yoshizumi T, et al. A simple and accurate formula to estimate left hepatic graft volume in living-donor adult liver transplantation. Transplantation 2004;77:1571–5.
17. Winter TC, Nghiem HV, Freeny PC, et al. Hepatic arterial anatomy: demonstration of normal supply and vascular variants with three dimensional CT angiography. Radiographics 1995;15:771–80.
18. Barr ML, Belghiti J, Villamil FG, et al. A report of the Vancouver Forum on the care of the live organ donor: lung, liver, pancreas, and intestine data and medical guidelines. Transplantation 2006;81:1373–85.
19. Botha JF, Campos BD, Johanning J, et al. Endovascular closure of a hemi portocaval shunt after small-for-size adult-to-adult left lobe living donor liver transplantation. Liver Transpl 2009;15:1671–5.
20. Hwang S, Lee SG, Lee YJ, et al. Lessons learned from 1000 living donor liver transplantations in a single center: how to make living donations safe. Liver Transpl 2006;12:920–7.
21. Taketomi A, Kayashima H, Soejima Y, et al. Donor risk in adult-to-adult living donor liver transplantation: impact of left lobe graft. Transplantation 2009;87: 445–50.

22. Umeshita K, Fujiwara K, Kiyosawa K, et al. Operative morbidity of living liver donors in Japan. Lancet 2003;362:687–90.
23. Iida T, Ogura Y, Oike F, et al. Surgery-related morbidity in living donors for liver transplantation. Transplantation 2010;89:1276–82.
24. Lo CM. Complications and long-term outcome of living liver donors: a survey of 1508 cases in five Asian centers. Transplantation 2003;75(Suppl 3):S12–5.
25. Marubashi S, Nagano H, Wada H, et al. Donor hepatectomy for living donor liver transplantation: learning steps and surgical outcome. Dig Dis Sci 2011;56: 2482–90.
26. Ghobrial RM, Freise CE, Trotter JF, et al. Donor morbidity after living donation for liver transplantation. Gastroenterology 2008;135:468–76.
27. Troisi R, Cammu G, Militerno G, et al. Modulation of portal graft inflow: a necessity in adult living-donor liver transplantation? Ann Surg 2003;237:429–36.
28. Troisi R, Ricciardi S, Smeets P, et al. Effects of hemi-portocaval shunts for inflow modulation on the outcome of small-for-size grafts in living donor liver transplantation. Am J Transplant 2005;5:1397–404.
29. Yamada T, Tanaka K, Uryuhara K, et al. Selective hemi-portocaval shunt based on portal vein pressure for small-for-size graft in adult living donor liver transplantation. Am J Transplant 2008;8:847–53.
30. Botha JF, Langnas AN, Campos BD, et al. Left lobe adult-to-adult living donor liver transplantation: small grafts and hemi-portocaval shunts in the prevention of small-for-size syndrome. Liver Transpl 2010;16:649–57.
31. Ogura Y, Hori T, El Moghazy WM, et al. Portal pressure <15 mm of Hg is a key for successful adult living donor liver transplantation utilizing smaller grafts than before. Liver Transpl 2010;16:718–28.
32. Ikegami T, Shirabe K, Soejima Y, et al. Strategies for successful left-lobe living donor liver transplantation in 250 consecutive adult cases in a single center. J Am Coll Surg 2013;216:353–62.
33. Kawasaki S, Makuuchi M, Matsunami H, et al. Living related liver transplantation in adults. Ann Surg 1998;227:269–74.
34. Shimada M, Shiotani S, Ninomiya M, et al. Characteristics of liver grafts in living-donor adult liver transplantation: comparison between right- and left-lobe grafts. Arch Surg 2002;137:1174–9.
35. Soejima Y, Shirabe K, Taketomi A, et al. Left lobe living donor liver transplantation in adults. Am J Transplant 2012;12:1877–85.
36. Soejima Y, Taketomi A, Yoshizumi T, et al. Feasibility of left-lobe living donor liver transplantation between adults: An 8-years, single center experience of 107 cases. Am J Transplant 2006;6:1004–11.
37. Ikegami T, Masuda Y, Ohno Y, et al. Prognosis of adult patients transplanted with liver grafts <35% of their standard liver volume. Liver Transpl 2009;15:1622–30.
38. Ishizaki Y, Kawasaki S, Sugo H, et al. Left lobe adult-to-adult living donor liver transplantation: Should portal inflow modulation be added? Liver Transpl 2012; 18:305–14.
39. Saidi RF, Jabbour N, Li Y, et al. Is left lobe adult-to-adult living donor liver transplantation ready for widespread use? The US experience (1998-2010). HPB (Oxford) 2012;14:455–60.

General Surgery Considerations in the Era of Mechanical Circulatory Assist Devices

Limael E. Rodriguez, MD, Erik E. Suarez, MD,
Matthias Loebe, MD, PhD, Brian A. Bruckner, MD*

KEYWORDS

- LVAD • Noncardiac surgery • Left ventricular assist device • General surgery
- Mechanical circulatory support

KEY POINTS

- Much of the success of left ventricular assist devices (LVAD) can be attributed to the second-generation HeartMate II (Thoratec, Pleasanton, CA), which is the most commonly used device to date.
- The key element introduced in second- generation devices was an internal rotor in the axial path of flow that was suspended via blood-immersed bearings (ie, the rotor is in direct contact with blood flow).
- The latest generation of LVADs is currently undergoing clinical trials worldwide. Developers have focused on improving on the limitations of the second- generation with emphasis on further enhancing efficiency, decreasing complications, and increasing ease of implantability.
- To understand the optimal surgical candidate better in the presence of an LVAD, one must understand the planned strategy afforded to the recipient at the time of implantation. This will allow the surgeon to understand the logistical and clinical characteristics of the LVAD patient population better.
- It is highly recommended that a cardiovascular anesthesiologist perform the anesthesia in the perioperative period and that the operation be performed in a cardiovascular surgery suite unless the procedure requires a special suite for completion.
- Bleeding and thromboembolism are serious adverse events that have been associated with the use of LVADs. In the setting of noncardiac surgeries, this has the potential to affect surgical outcomes, especially when the surgery is emergent or classified as a major intervention.
- Clinical management of a patient with an LVAD is also an excellent example of the multidisciplinary approach of care that is undoubtedly the future of medicine.

Financial Disclosure and Conflict of Interest: The authors have nothing to disclose.
Department of Cardiovascular Surgery, Methodist DeBakey Heart & Vascular Center, Houston Methodist Hospital, 6550 Fannin Street, Suite 1401, Houston, TX 77030, USA
* Corresponding author.
E-mail address: babruckner@houstonmethodist.org

Surg Clin N Am 93 (2013) 1343–1357
http://dx.doi.org/10.1016/j.suc.2013.08.004
surgical.theclinics.com

INTRODUCTION

Now that more than 6800 left ventricular assist devices (LVAD) have been surgically implanted worldwide,[1] it is evident that a new age of heart failure management is being entered into. With an estimated 5 million patients with heart failure in the United States alone, and up to 550,000 new patients diagnosed yearly,[2] this therapy has become a welcome addition to heart failure treatment options. Much of the LVAD success can be attributed to the second-generation HeartMate II (Thoratec, Pleasanton, CA, USA), which is the most commonly used device to date. Landmark studies, such as the HeartMate II Destination Therapy trial, have demonstrated the significant survival benefits of this device when compared with medical therapy alone. These significant survival benefits have led to an exponential rate of implantation over the last 6 years, with almost 40% of the implants strategically placed as a long-term destination therapy (DT) without plans for transplantation.[3] The current survival rates with second-generation continuous-flow pumps exceed 80% at 1 year and 70% at 2 years.[1] Clinicians in noncardiac specialties are now encountering this patient population with increased frequency. General surgery is no exception, as various literature reports have been published over the past 2 decades describing experiences with mechanical support. In this review, generations of LVAD devices are discussed briefly and the current implications of the LVAD patient for general surgery are analyzed.

HISTORY
First Generation: Arrival of the LVAD

The first generation of implantable devices pump blood via pulsation, hence the term pulsatile pump. The HeartMate I (Thoratec Corp), Thoratec PVAD (Thoratec Corp), and Novacor N100 (World Heart, Inc, Oakland, CA, USA) are the devices that represent this first-generation group. Implantation requires a median sternotomy with the pump located intra-abdominally (**Fig. 1**). The pump size is significantly larger than newer generation models and requires an extra air displacement chamber pocket. Intrinsically, first-generation devices have large tissue and blood contacting surfaces, as well as multiple moving parts.[4] Long-term oral anticoagulation therapy with warfarin is generally recommended.

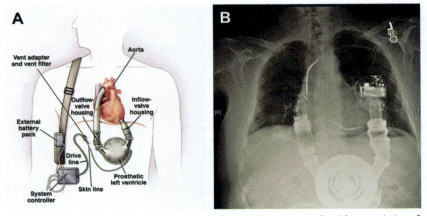

Fig. 1. First-generation LVAD. (*A*) Diagram of HeartMate I. Used with permission from Thoratec Corporation, Pleasanton, CA. (*B*) Chest radiograph of implanted HeartMate I.

Because long-term support was the objective, the high risk of infection, thrombus formation, and blood trauma were significant complications that needed to be addressed.[4–8] From a practical point of view, comfort/ease of use for patients and mechanical durability of the pump were also not optimal for long-term use. Despite these limitations, the first-generation LVAD did result in significant improvement in survival. This improvement was illustrated in the end points of the landmark REMATCH trial, which showed a 46% decrease in death from any cause and a 1-year survival of 52% with LVAD versus 25% with medical therapy alone.[9]

Second Generation: Improved and Established Outcomes

The second-generation LVAD developers focused on decreasing size and complications, while improving efficiency and durability. To accomplish these goals, researchers focused on the development and principles of continuous flow pumps. The HeartMate II (Thoratec Corp) (**Fig. 2**), Jarvik 2000 (Jarvik Heart, New York, NY, USA), and Micromed DeBakey (MicroMed Cardiovascular, Houston, TX, USA) highlight this class of devices.

The key element introduced in second-generation devices was an internal rotor in the axial path of flow that was suspended via blood-immersed bearings (ie, the rotor is in direct contact with blood flow).[10] The benefit of this design was further reduction of pro-thrombotic sites, optimization of efficiency that was previously hampered by multiple moving parts, and a significant decrease in pump size. Efficiency was further enhanced with elimination of the reservoir chamber and inflow/outflow valves. The HeartMate II pump is placed in a preperitoneal pocket, or occasionally is placed intra-abdominally, with the driveline exiting the abdomen (see **Fig. 2**).[11] Benchmark mechanical life of second-generation LVADs is estimated to be at least 5 years, but longer support has been well documented.[12] Long-term anticoagulation is required and in accordance with the recommendations of specific device manufacturers.[13,14] In 2007, the HeartMate II bridge to transplant (BTT) trial became another landmark study for implantable LVADs. It showed survival rates of 75% at 6 months and 68%

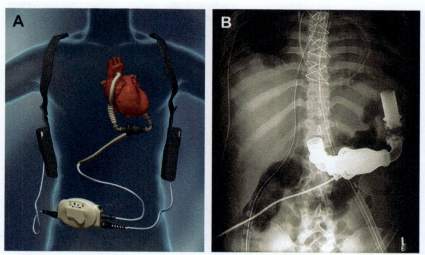

Fig. 2. Second-generation LVAD. (*A*) Diagram of HeartMate II LVAD. (*B*) Chest radiograph of implanted HeartMate II. Images used with permission from Thoratec Corporation, Pleasanton, CA.

at 1 year, with significantly improved quality of life and functional capacity.[15,16] This success led to the HeartMate II DT trial, which demonstrated significantly increased survival 2 years post implantation when compared to HeartMate I.[12]

Third Generation: Size, Efficiency, and Durability Optimized

The latest generation of LVADs is currently undergoing clinical trials worldwide. Developers have focused on improving on the limitations of the second- generation with emphasis on further enhancing efficiency, decreasing complications, and increasing ease of implantability. The DuraHeart (Terumo Heart, Ann Arbor, MI, USA), HeartWare HVAD (HeartWare International, Framingham, MA, USA), Incor (Berlin Heart, Berlin, Germany), Levacor (World Heart Inc, Salt Lake City, UT, USA), and the future HeartMate III (Thoratec Corp) highlight this class of devices. Leading the group is the HeartWare HVAD (**Fig. 3**) (recently FDA approved), which has a smaller pump design that can be implanted intrapericardically.

GENERAL SURGERY CONSIDERATIONS
Overview

A patient with an implanted LVAD may often be perceived as a high-risk surgical candidate. Surgeons unfamiliar with the LVAD profile often think there to be advanced heart failure, which may result in a premature decision to recommend nonsurgical therapy. Over the past 18 years, various reports have demonstrated that patients with LVADs can have very successful outcomes in most elective noncardiac surgeries (NCS). Of particular interest has been the intraoperative management of these patients while they undergo the NCS procedures. Several studies have examined the surgical, anesthetic, and logistic factors that are important in the successful intraoperative management of these patients. These same studies have helped shape the way clinicians approach LVAD surgical candidates in the perioperative period. In this section, the recommendations made to date are reviewed.

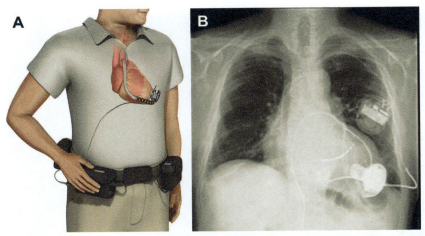

Fig. 3. Third-generation HVAD. (*A*) Diagram of HeartWare HVAD. Used with permission from HeartWare International, Framingham, MA. (*B*) Chest radiograph of implanted HeartWare HVAD. (*From* Haeck ML, Hoogslag GE, Rodrigo SF, et al. Treatment options in endstage heart failure: where to go from here? Neth Heart J 2012;20(4):172; with permission.)

Patient Selection

To understand the optimal surgical candidate better in the presence of an LVAD, one must understand the planned strategy afforded to the recipient at the time of implantation. This planned strategy will allow the surgeon to understand the logistical and clinical characteristics of the LVAD patient population better. An LVAD recipient can be broadly differentiated into 2 planned strategies: BTT or DT. This differentiation is a critical question that should be asked when inquiring about the patient's LVAD status. The former, BTT, allows the clinician to understand that the patient did not have any major transplant contraindications (ie, renal dysfunction, current smoker, or other comorbidities). This BTT in turn allowed the patient to meet criteria for cardiac transplantation candidacy. The BTT group, along with the subgroup known as bridge to transplant candidacy, accounts for 65% of currently used LVAD strategies.[1] An excellent example of a transition between bridge to transplant candidacy and BTT is the concomitant use of bariatric weight loss surgery with LVAD implantation in patients who are morbidly obese with end-stage heart disease.[17] The hope is that, with sustained weight loss and the survival benefits of the LVAD, the patient can later become a candidate for cardiac transplantation.

In contrast, DT therapy patients have modifiable and/or nonmodifiable risk factors that reserved the patient from being considered for a cardiac transplantation.[1] The most common nonmodifiable factors are advanced age and other comorbidities. The most common modifiable risk factors are renal dysfunction, high body mass index, and secondary pulmonary hypertension. Thus, knowing the LVAD strategy can open the door for many questions about the patient's current state.

Equally important are the risk factors for early death that were reported in the fifth annual Interagency Registry for Mechanically Assisted Circulatory Support (INTERMACS) report, the North American registry that has followed all LVADs implanted since 2006.[1] A major contribution of INTERMACS has been the delineation of risk factors for morbidity and mortality. For instance, age, high blood urea nitrogen, DT therapy, and right heart failure (with concomitant ascites) were all cited as very significant constant hazard risk factors for death. History of previous cardiac surgery is the most significant constant risk factor. The early hazard risk factors were cited to be age, high body surface area, previous cardiac surgical intervention, and high blood urea nitrogen. Moreover, the most significant early hazard risk factor was the patients INTERMACS level score (ranging from 1–7), which is a calculated scale that considers all pre-implant risk factors before receiving LVAD (**Table 1**). A lower number affords a worse status, with INTERMACS 1 demarcating cardiogenic shock at the time of LVAD implant planning. Most patients scores range between 2 and 5, as most ventricular assist device (VAD) surgeons shy away from implanting the very high-risk group with a score of 1. Independent studies have supported the validity of the scoring system to assess patient profiles and predict the risk of complications.[18]

Surgical Planning

As describe above, the profile of a patient implanted with an LVAD has serious implications that a surgeon must acknowledge. In turn, additional planning and resources are critical to ensuring safety when an NCS procedure is being considered. Firstenberg and colleagues[19] were one of the first groups to publish guidelines for the management of patients requiring NCS in the setting of an LVAD. In their report, a critical aspect of care was the collaboration of the noncardiac surgeons with the designated VAD team, which includes the adult cardiac surgery attending, cardiovascular (CV) anesthesiologist, CV nurse, perfusionist, and specialty pharmacist (**Fig. 4**). It is highly

Table 1 INTERMACS MCS[a] early and constant hazard risk factors for death				
	Early Hazard		**Constant Hazard**	
Risk Factors for Death	**Hazard Ratio**	**P Value**	**Hazard Ratio**	**P Value**
Demographics				
Age (older)	1.69	<.0001	—	—
Body mass index (higher)	1.47	<.0001	—	—
Clinical status				
Ventilator	1.65	.009	—	—
History of stroke	1.69	.009	—	—
INTERMACS level 1	2.45	<.0001	—	—
INTERMACS level 2	1.89	.0004	1.30	.003
Destination therapy	—	—	1.25	.01
Noncardiac systems				
Diabetes	—	—	1.22	.02
Creatinine (higher)	—	—	1.1	.008
Dialysis	2.22	.002	—	—
Blood urea nitrogen (higher)	1.10	<.0001	—	—
Right heart dysfunction				
RVAD in same operation	3.73	<.0001	—	—
Right atrial pressure (higher)	1.36	.002	—	—
Bilirubin (higher)	1.08	<.0001	—	—
Ascites	—	—	1.32	.05
Surgical complexities				
History of cardiac surgery	—	—	1.50	<.0001
Concomitant cardiac surgery	1.34	.02	—	—

Abbreviations: BiVAD, biventricular assist device; MCS, mechanical circulatory support; RVAD, right ventricular assist device.

[a] Implants: June 2006 to June 2012, Adult Primary Continuous-Flow LVADs and BiVADS, DT, and BTT (n = 5436).

Adapted from Kirklin JK, Naftel DC, Kormos RL, et al. Fifth INTERMACS annual report: risk factor analysis from more than 6000 mechanical circulatory support patients. J Heart Lung Transplant 2013;32(2):141–56.

recommended that a CV anesthesiologist perform the anesthesia in the perioperative period and that the operation be performed in a CV surgery suite unless the procedure requires a special suite for completion. Arterial line monitoring and/or a central venous catheter is typically required to monitor blood pressure and cardiac output during major procedures that place patients at risk for hemodynamic instability.[20] For minor operations, Doppler blood pressure monitoring is acceptable. Minimally invasive surgical approaches are intuitively preferred, particularly for intra-abdominal procedures. However, care must be taken when placing ports or making surgical incisions, as the driveline and pump are potentially located intra-abdominally. Also critical is that intra-abdominal insufflation should be kept at the minimal level needed to provide adequate surgical exposure, as LVAD function extremely depends on preload. If preload is inhibited, the device may collapse the left ventricle due to lack of blood to pump, placing the patient at high risk for a serious event.[20–22] Although treatment of such an event is straightforward, strict vigilance of the preload and other VAD parameters is critical, which is the reason a perfusionist is required during the entirety of the

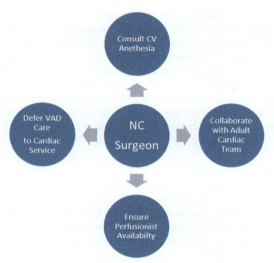

Fig. 4. Key collaborations for noncardiac surgeons.

case. Postoperative care requires admission to the adult cardiac surgery service for monitoring and care of VAD-associated events (see **Fig. 4** for an overview of the continuity of care).

GENERAL SURGERY CONSULTS AND OPERATIONS

As the implantation of LVADs has exponentially increased over the past 10 years, so has the frequency of NCS consultation and resultant operations. This increase has forced general surgeons to become part of the continuum of care and adjust to unique characteristics of this patient population. A review of multiple literature reports since 1995 has shown that almost all common general surgery consults have been experienced in the LVAD population (**Table 2**).[23–31] The most common operations performed were of intra-abdominal pathologic abnormality. These procedures range from cholecystectomy to appendectomy and from exploratory laparotomy to large and small bowel resections. Tracheostomy was also frequently cited as a common procedure. Urologic, gynecologic, orthopedic, neurosurgical, dental, and ENT procedures have also been frequently reported. NCS consultations specifically related to

| Table 2 | | |
| General surgery operations reported in LVAD patients | | |
General Surgery Operations	**No. Reported**	**% Overall**
Tracheostomy	27	20
Abdominal[a]	65	47
Hernias/hemorrhoids	15	11
Skin/debridement	13	9
Vascular	18	13
Total	138	100

[a] Intra-abdominal procedures that involved gastrum, small/large bowel, biliary, spleen, or abscesses.
Data from Refs.[24–27,30–33]

the device (pump pocket infection, driveline infection) have expectedly decreased in frequency. This decrease has been attributed to the design improvements, better patient selection, increased provider experience, and improved follow-up care with the specialized VAD team.[23] In terms of design, the second-generation pumps are markedly smaller and less bulky, minimizing required intra-abdominal compartmentalization. This limitation was a major concern of the first-generation pumps, which frequently required surgical debridement and cleaning of pump pocket infections. Thus, second-generation LVADs are more likely to present as outpatient referral with elective surgical problems common for age and natural history.[24]

OUTCOMES

Multiple retrospective reviews have ascertained the outcomes of NCS in the LVAD patient. For the most part, the studies demonstrate that reasonable results can be attained (**Table 3**). However, complication rates tend to be higher when compared with the general population. Moreover, routine perioperative care and special considerations are necessary in LVAD recipients who require surgical therapy. Goldstein and colleagues[25] were the first to demonstrate successful outcomes of NCS in the setting of the LVAD. Unfortunately, from a device point of view, these retrospective articles are rapidly becoming outdated as all cases were performed with original, first-generation pulsatile devices. Nevertheless, the authors were able to draw conclusions regarding the basic principles of what should be expected in the perioperative period. A major contribution was the highlighted importance of cardiac preload management, as LVAD function significantly depends on this factor. Goldstein and colleagues elucidated the need for strict vigilance of body positioning and reported that proper hydration throughout the procedure as an effective measure to treat positional preload changes. Following this protocol, the intraoperative courses were uncomplicated and none of the patients required significant vasopressor support or blood product transfusion to maintain blood pressure. This study also proposed that an individual from the operating team (surgeon, anesthesiologist, or nurse) familiar with the device should be available immediately if needed during the intra/perioperative period. This availability of a surgical team member was thought to be a critical factor if good outcomes were to be expected.

In most literature reports to date, bleeding events have been cited as the most common postoperative major complication in NCS cases. Schmid and colleagues[26] demonstrated that more than half of their patients had some type of complication, usually a hemorrhagic event and extended output from drains. They postulated that this was the result of clinical reluctance to lower anticoagulation therapy, which primarily entails warfarin, aspirin, and heparin as a measure to reduce thrombotic events. They concluded that anticoagulation therapy needed to be managed in a more restricted fashion, as this resulted in better outcomes and less incidence of bleeding events. The key limitation of this study is that 100% of the patients had a pulsatile LVAD, which have been rarely implanted since 2006 due to second-generation pumps.

In another study, Brown and colleagues[27] demonstrated the significance of the patient profile in the NCS preoperative period. They showed that patients who underwent NCS during the same admission as their VAD implant had a 40% survival to discharge; this was a significant mortality difference when compared with the 75% survival to discharge seen in patients who returned for an elective procedure at a subsequent visit. This disparity demonstrated that 2 distinct patient profiles existed in which the need for NCS intervention in the early LVAD implantation period correlates with a higher risk for poor outcome. This poor outcome may be attributed to the generalized inflammatory response in all patients undergoing major cardiac surgery. It has been well documented that cardiac surgery provokes a vigorous inflammatory response that causes the patient to remain in critical condition in the immediate post-operative period.[28] In a 2003 report from the Society of Thoracic Surgeons database, coronary artery bypass grafting had 30-day mortality and major composite morbidity rates of 3% and 13%, respectively.[29] The cause of this high-risk period is likely multi-factorial, including cardiopulmonary bypass –initiated hemodynamic changes, subop-timal organ perfusion during cardiopulmonary bypass, and anti-inflammatory immune responses in the perioperative period. Thus, similar to a classic coronary artery bypass grafting, the implantation of an LVAD causes major hemodynamic and immunomod-ulatory changes that entails an extended stabilization period.

In the largest study to date, Stehlik and colleagues[30] reviewed data on 37 patients who received a total of 59 elective surgical procedures. Most procedures (68%) were common general surgery interventions that ranged from cholecystectomy, to inguinal/ventral hernia repair, to colon resection. They reported that 75% were not systemat-ically on oral anticoagulation at the time of surgery. The majority (>95%) of the patient strategies presented as either BTT or DT. All but 3 of the 59 cases were performed in the VAD implantation operating suite. Most cases were considered to be nonemergent and 12 were classified as emergent. There were no deaths in the immediate postop-erative time and the 30-day mortality was 12% overall. Moreover, of the mortalities, 6% were from nonemergent surgeries and 33% from emergent surgeries. Of the 18 pa-tients who had VADs implanted as a BTT, 6 patients were discharged without compli-cations and 8 underwent cardiac transplantation in the same hospital stay. The study concluded that elective NCS had very good outcomes as long as the procedure was nonemergent and in close collaboration with the VAD team. The only limitation of this report was that most VADs implanted were pulsatile devices.

More recent reports have studied NCS in the second-generation axial flow LVAD population. In a smaller report by Ahmed and colleagues,[31] no morbidities or compli-cations in first 30 days postoperatively were reported in patients who had extended times with an implant. Their subjects had an average LVAD implantation time of 500 days. In turn, they demonstrated that DT patients who already had more than 1 year of implantation with the second-generation HeartMate II device can have very good outcomes. The study by Morgan and colleagues[32] showed similar out-comes in patients with the HeartMate II LVAD. This study included 20 patients who underwent a total of 25 NCS. They clinically classified the cases as emergent and non-emergent, with further subclassification of major and minor procedures. The major NCS included cholecystectomy, bilateral salpingo-oophorectomy, small bowel obstruction, and colon resections. Morgan and colleagues reported no perioperative deaths, thromboembolic complications, or device malfunctions. They demonstrated a significant incidence (36%) of bleeding requiring transfusion of packed red blood cells, which was present in almost half the patients classified as undergoing major sur-gery. All bleeding complications occurred in patients on preoperative dual anticoagu-lation (warfarin and aspirin). They also demonstrated that preoperative warfarin use and high international normalized ratio (INR) were the predictors of bleeding in the transfusion group. They concluded that bleeding events were likely due to anticoagu-lation and that lowering the preoperative anticoagulation goals may reduce the incidence of perioperative bleeding.

ANTICOAGULATION

As mentioned above, bleeding and thromboembolism are serious adverse events that have been associated with the use of LVADs. In the setting of NCS, this has the

Table 3
Literature reports on NCS in LVAD population

Study	VAD Type	Patient No. (Mean Age)	Total NCS Procedures	TWI PreOp (d)	Results	Complications	Conclusions
Goldstein et al,[25] 1995	Pulse-100%	8 (52.7)	12	68 + 35	All VADS pulsatile; no surgery-associated morbidity	Hypotension with positional change in 4/8 patients	Patient positioning, device limitations, fluid and inotropic management will help improve outcomes
Schmid et al,[26] 2001	Pulse-100%	14 (44 + 15)	14	53 + 57	All VADs pulsatile; half of NCS were performed within 30 d of VAD implant	Complications in 57%; mostly bleeding	Recommended postponement of anticoagulation; elective NCS is feasible; emergent remains difficult
Garatti et al,[33] 2009	Axial-73% Pulse-27%	11 (52)	12	58.7 + 45.6	90.9% of patients required blood transfusions; no early perioperative mortality	2 patients died of intracranial hemorrhages and multiorgan failure at 45- and 13-d postop	Intraoperative coagulation management is key to safety; NCS is feasible and safe
Brown et al,[27] 2009	Axial-33% Pulse-29% Ext-38%	25 (55)	27	199 + 181	Perioperative survival 100%; 28-d survival 64%	Bleeding 48%; infection 33%	NCS is feasible and safe; bleeding complications were common

Stehlik et al,[30] 2009	Pulse->90%	37 (56 + 16)	59	30-d mortality 12%	Bleeding 10%; abdominal re-exploration in 20%	VAD management in postop period in critically ill patients; NCS is feasible if management includes VAD team
Ahmed et al,[31] 2012	Axial-85%	6 (60.8)	6	No 30-d mortality	None reported	NCS can be performed safely in DT patients
Morgan et al,[32] 2012	Axial-100%	20 (50.1 + 12.7)	25	No perioperative deaths; no significant long-term survival difference; higher bleeding incidence in major surgeries	Need for PRBCs 36%	Reasonable to lower or normalize INR preoperatively
McKellar et al,[24] 2012	Axial-81%	27 (60 + 13)	28	30-d survival 81%	None	Outcomes better in 2nd-generation devices

Abbreviations: PRBCs, packed red blood cells; TWI, time with implant (days).
Data from Refs.[24–27,30–33]

potential to affect surgical outcomes, especially when the surgery is emergent or classified as a major intervention. Fortunately, much of the NCS postoperative anticoagulation management can be addressed by studies that have delineated optimal anticoagulation and the 2013 International Society of Heart and Lung Transplantation guidelines for mechanical assist devices.[13–15,20,33–35] Key recommendations for preoperative anticoagulation management depend on the bleeding risk for a specific noncardiac procedure and the severity of the disease process at clinical presentation. For nonemergency procedures, warfarin and aspirin (dual therapy) may be continued if the risk of bleeding associated with the procedure is low. For emergency procedures, warfarin may need to be rapidly reversed with fresh frozen plasma or prothrombin complex concentrate. Administration of vitamin K may be considered, but slower onset of action must be taken into consideration. If anticoagulation therapy needs to be stopped, dual therapy should be held accordingly based on the type of procedure being undertaken and risk of bleeding. While not taking warfarin, bridging with heparin may be considered.

Initial recommendations for postoperative anticoagulation for the HeartMate II and most LVADs involved intravenous heparin followed by aspirin and warfarin, targeting an INR of 2.5 to 3.5. However, landmark revisions were made in 2009 after Boyle and colleagues[13] demonstrated high rates of bleeding and low rates of thrombosis. Their study concluded that an INR of less than 1.5 was associated with higher thrombotic events, and bleeding incidence was significantly increased with INRs greater than 2.5. Therefore, it was concluded that heparinization increases the risk of prolonged bleeding, and that postoperative therapy with aspirin and warfarin targeting an INR between 1.5 and 2.5 was reasonable. However, continuation of heparin may be considered while waiting for the target INR goal, and dual therapy may be resumed when risk of surgical bleeding is deemed acceptable (ie, output from drains is minimal). Therefore, in the early postoperative period, the patient's anticoagulation status should be checked frequently and accordingly. The use of other antiplatelet agents may be considered, but is not the standard of care.

SUMMARY

An exciting time in medicine is being entered into in which technology plays a critical role for treating diseases that were at one time considered intractable. A decade ago, most patients with end-stage heart failure were treated with medical therapy, resulting in a 1-year survival that was unacceptably low (49%) when compared with today's standards.[36] Current 2-year survival rates when treated with LVAD are approximately 70%, thus providing a major patient population with a proven long-term therapeutic strategy. Moreover, improved LVAD design has resulted in fewer complications directly related to the device and more common noncardiac pathologic abnormalities unrelated to the device are presenting clinically.

Clinical management of a patient with an LVAD is also an excellent example of the multidisciplinary approach of care that is undoubtedly the future of medicine. Most guidelines and reports recommend full collaboration between the VAD team, transplant surgeons, heart failure cardiologist, CV anesthesiologist, and noncardiac surgeon (see **Fig. 4**). As is the case for most critical disease states, this multidisciplinary approach translates into optimized patient safety and satisfaction, and improved outcomes.

In closing, patients with LVADs are increasingly requiring consultation and intervention from noncardiac surgeons. As second-generation devices have become the standard, they will be the device encountered for years to come. The design has excellent long-term results; thus, patients will more frequently present as outpatients with common elective surgical problems. General surgeons should be prepared to deal with the problems that are characteristic of this patient population. The ability to understand the logistical nature of the strategy used (BTT or DT), assess the clinical status of the patient at presentation, and collaborate with VAD specialists are all critical components of care that will improve this new and exciting experience.

ACKNOWLEDGMENTS

The authors thank Amanda Hodgson, PhD, for critical reading of the article.

REFERENCES

1. Kirklin JK, Naftel DC, Kormos RL, et al. Fifth INTERMACS annual report: risk factor analysis from more than 6,000 mechanical circulatory support patients. J Heart Lung Transplant 2013;32(2):141–56.
2. Hunt SA, Abraham WT, Chin MH, et al. 2009 Focused update incorporated into the ACC/AHA 2005 Guidelines for the Diagnosis and Management of Heart Failure in Adults A Report of the American College of Cardiology Foundation/American Heart Association Task Force on Practice Guidelines Developed in Collaboration With the International Society for Heart and Lung Transplantation. J Am Coll Cardiol 2009;53(15):e1–90.
3. Kirklin JK, Naftel DC, Kormos RL, et al. The fourth INTERMACS annual report: 4,000 implants and counting. J Heart Lung Transplant 2012;31(2):117–26.
4. Goldstein DJ, Oz MC, Rose EA. Implantable left ventricular assist devices. N Engl J Med 1998;339(21):1522–33.
5. Farrar DJ, Bourque K, Dague CP, et al. Design features, developmental status, and experimental results with the HeartMate III centrifugal left ventricular assist system with a magnetically levitated rotor. ASAIO J 2007;53(3):310–5.
6. El-Banayosy A, Arusoglu L, Kizner L, et al. Novacor left ventricular assist system versus HeartMate vented electric left ventricular assist system as a long-term mechanical circulatory support device in bridging patients: a prospective study. J Thorac Cardiovasc Surg 2000;119(3):581–7.
7. Nicholson C, Paz JC. Total artificial heart and physical therapy management. Cardiopulm Phys Ther J 2010;21(2):13–21.
8. Frazier OH, Myers TJ, Radovancević B. The HeartMate left ventricular assist system. Overview and 12-year experience. Tex Heart Inst J 1998;25(4):265–71.
9. Rose EA, Gelijns AC, Moskowitz AJ, et al. Long-term use of a left ventricular assist device for end-stage heart failure. N Engl J Med 2001;345(20):1435–43.
10. Burke DJ, Burke E, Parsaie F, et al. The HeartMate II: design and development of a fully sealed axial flow left ventricular assist system. Artif Organs 2001;25(5): 380–5.
11. Slaughter MS. Long-term continuous flow left ventricular assist device support and end-organ function: prospects for destination therapy. J Card Surg 2010; 25(4):490–4.
12. Slaughter MS, Rogers JG, Milano CA, et al. Advanced heart failure treated with continuous-flow left ventricular assist device. N Engl J Med 2009;361(23): 2241–51.
13. Boyle AJ, Russell SD, Teuteberg JJ, et al. Low thromboembolism and pump thrombosis with the HeartMate II left ventricular assist device: analysis of outpatient anti-coagulation. J Heart Lung Transplant 2009;28(9):881–7.

14. John R, Kamdar F, Liao K, et al. Low thromboembolic risk for patients with the HeartMate II left ventricular assist device. J Thorac Cardiovasc Surg 2008; 136(5):1318-23.
15. Miller LW, Pagani FD, Russell SD, et al. Use of a continuous-flow device in patients awaiting heart transplantation. N Engl J Med 2007;357(9):885-96.
16. Popov AF, Hosseini MT, Zych B, et al. Clinical experience with HeartwAre left ventricular assist device in patients with end-stage heart failure. Ann Thorac Surg 2012;93(3):810-5.
17. Gill RS, Karmali S, Nagandran J, et al. Combined Ventricular Assist Device Placement With Adjustable Gastric Band (VAD-BAND): a promising new technique for morbidly obese patients awaiting potential cardiac transplantation. J Clin Med Res 2012;4(2):127-9.
18. Alba AC, Rao V, Ivanov J, et al. Usefulness of the INTERMACS scale to predict outcomes after mechanical assist device implantation. J Heart Lung Transplant 2009;28(8):827-33.
19. Firstenberg MS, Sai-Sudhakar C, Abel E, et al. Institutional guidelines for the care of the patient with a ventricular-assist device requiring non-cardiac surgery. Mech Circ Support 2011;2:5978.
20. Feldman D, Pamboukian SV, Teuteberg JJ, et al. The 2013 International Society for Heart and Lung Transplantation Guidelines for mechanical circulatory support: executive summary. J Heart Lung Transplant 2013;32(2):157-87.
21. Kirkpatrick JN. Echocardiographic evaluation of ventricular support devices. In: St John Sutton M, Wiegers SE, editors. Practical echocardiography: echocardiography in heart failure. Philadelphia: Elsevier Saunders; 2012. p. 181-94.
22. Moazami N, Fukamachi K, Kobayashi M, et al. Axial and centrifugal continuous-flow rotary pumps: a translation from pump mechanics to clinical practice. J Heart Lung Transplant 2013;32(1):1-11.
23. Schaffer JM, Allen JG, Weiss ES, et al. Infectious complications after pulsatile-flow and continuous-flow left ventricular assist device implantation. J Heart Lung Transplant 2011;30(2):164-74.
24. McKellar SH, Morris DS, Mauermann WJ, et al. Evolution of general surgical problems in patients with left ventricular assist devices. Surgery 2012;152(5):896-902.
25. Goldstein DJ, Mullis SL, Delphin ES, et al. Noncardiac surgery in long-term implantable left ventricular assist-device recipients. Ann Surg 1995;222(2): 203-7.
26. Schmid C, Wilhelm M, Dietl KH, et al. Noncardiac surgery in patients with long term left ventricular assist devices. Surgery 2001;129(4):440-4.
27. Brown JB, Hallinan WM, Massey HT, et al. Does the need for noncardiac surgery during ventricular assist device therapy impact clinical outcome? Surgery 2009; 146(4):627-33 [discussion: 633-4].
28. Loebe M, Koster A, Sänger S, et al. Inflammatory response after implantation of a left ventricular assist device: comparison between the axial flow MicroMed DeBakey VAD and the pulsatile Novacor device. ASAIO J 2001;47(3):272-4.
29. Shroyer AL, Coombs LP, Peterson ED, et al. The Society of Thoracic Surgeons: 30-day operative mortality and morbidity risk models. Ann Thorac Surg 2003; 75(6):1856-64 [discussion: 1864-5].
30. Stehlik J, Nelson DM, Kfoury AG, et al. Outcome of noncardiac surgery in patients with ventricular assist devices. Am J Cardiol 2009;103(5):709-12.
31. Ahmed M, Le H, Aranda JM Jr, et al. Elective noncardiac surgery in patients with left ventricular assist devices. J Card Surg 2012;27(5):639-42.

32. Morgan JA, Paone G, Nemeh HW, et al. Non-cardiac surgery in patients on long-term left ventricular assist device support. J Heart Lung Transplant 2012;31(7): 757–63.
33. Garatti A, Bruschi G, Colombo T, et al. Noncardiac surgical procedures in patient supported with long-term implantable left ventricular assist device. Am J Surg 2009;197(6):710–4.
34. Allen SJ, Sidebotham D. Postoperative care and complications after ventricular assist device implantation. Best Pract Res Clin Anaesthesiol 2012;26(2):231–46.
35. Slaughter MS, Pagani FD, Rogers JG, et al. Clinical management of continuous-flow left ventricular assist devices in advanced heart failure. J Heart Lung Transplant 2010;29(Suppl 4):S1–39.
36. Pamboukianm SV, Tallaj JA, Brown RN, et al. Comparison of observed survival after ventricular assist device placement versus predicted survival without assist device using the Seattle heart failure model. ASAIO J 2012;58(2):93–7.

Bariatric Surgery and End-Stage Organ Failure

Nabil Tariq, MD[a], Linda W. Moore, MS, RD, CCRP[b],
Vadim Sherman, MD, FRCSC[a],*

KEYWORDS

- Kidney transplantation • Liver transplantation • Bariatric surgery • Obesity

KEY POINTS

- Morbid obesity increases the risk of complications and allograft failure in transplant patients.
- Bariatric surgery is both safe and effective in patients with chronic kidney disease and end-stage renal disease, and helps patients become eligible for transplant based on body mass index.
- Bariatric surgery does not affect postoperative immunosuppressant dosing regimens.
- Bariatric surgery in patients with liver disease has been shown to be safe and effective, although this population remains at high risk, especially in the setting of portal hypertension.
- Sleeve gastrectomy may become increasingly utilized in pretransplant and posttransplant patients, as it has been shown to result in low complication rates and excellent weight loss, and retains intestinal continuity.

SCOPE OF THE PROBLEM

Access to organ transplantation is affected by obesity, especially morbid obesity, because of the increased risks associated with surgical procedures, the risk of graft loss, wound complications, a higher risk for new-onset diabetes following transplantation, and a greater risk of death.[1–4] In addition to these objective measures, several technical factors increase the complexity of surgery in patients with morbid obesity. To this end, most transplant centers have established criteria related specifically to body mass, and will therefore prevent patients whose body mass index (BMI; calculated as weight in kilograms divided by height in meters squared, ie, kg/m^2) is greater than 40 to be listed for transplantation. For these patients to become candidates for

[a] Bariatric and Metabolic Surgery Center, Department of Surgery, Houston Methodist Hospital, 6550 Fannin Street, SM 1661, Houston, TX 77030, USA; [b] Research Programs, Department of Surgery, Houston Methodist Hospital Physician Organization, 6550 Fannin Street, SM 1661, Houston, TX 77030, USA
* Corresponding author.
E-mail address: vsherman@HoustonMethodist.org

Surg Clin N Am 93 (2013) 1359–1371
http://dx.doi.org/10.1016/j.suc.2013.08.006
0039-6109/13/$ – see front matter © 2013 Elsevier Inc. All rights reserved.

transplantation, weight loss is an absolute prerequisite to listing.[2] In general, morbid obesity and its many associated comorbidities have been shown to increase the risk of cardiovascular disease within the general population. In patients with chronic kidney disease (CKD), obesity has been shown to increase the incidence of cardiovascular disease and left ventricular hypertrophy,[2] and is associated with cardiovascular disease in epidemiologic studies.[5]

INCIDENCE OF OBESITY IN THE UNITED STATES, IN CKD, AND IN KIDNEY TRANSPLANTATION

The increase in obesity in the United States is a well-known fact.[6] In 2010, more than two-thirds of adults in the United States were overweight (BMI ≥25) or obese (BMI ≥30; **Fig. 1**). As the incidence of obesity has increased, so too has the incidence of several obesity-related comorbidities, specifically diabetes mellitus and hypertension. The result has been that all-cause mortality is increased in the normal population at higher grades of obesity.[7] In patients with kidney disease, the story parallels that of the normal United States population. In 1995, only 19.1% of incident patients with end-stage renal disease (ESRD) were overweight or obese, but by 2009 this proportion had risen to 37.9% of incident patients (**Fig. 2**).[8] Whereas the median BMI of patients presenting for treatment of ESRD is in the overweight category, BMI ranges include extreme obesity (BMI ≥40) for every ESRD modality, including transplantation (**Table 1**).

TREATMENTS FOR OBESITY IN KIDNEY DISEASE

The basis of weight loss involves a negative caloric balance whereby expenditure of calories is outweighed by intake. Limiting calories by 500 kcal/d will yield a weight loss of 0.5 kg/wk.[9] Unfortunately, simply instructing patients to eat less and exercise more is not an effective means for weight loss. Morbidly obese patients are generally 100 lb (45.4 kg) over their ideal weight, which means that a significant weight loss would require a significant amount of time. Compliance over this protracted time is the biggest limitation to conservative weight loss, and often leads to ineffective weight loss or

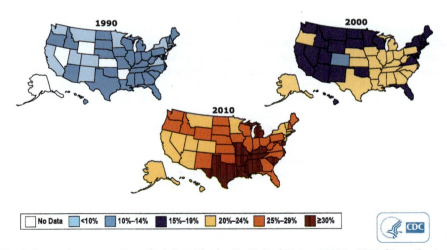

Fig. 1. Increasing proportion of adults with obesity, United States, 1990 to 2010. (*From* Centers for Disease Control and Prevention. Available at: http://www.cdc.gov/obesity/data/adult.html. Accessed August 15, 2013.)

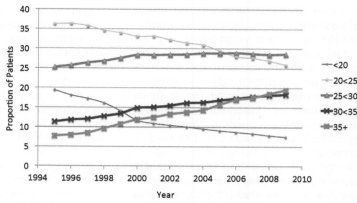

Fig. 2. Increasing proportion of incident ESRD patients with obesity, 1995 to 2009.

weight regain.[10] Efforts aimed at behavioral modification are more successful; however, in patients with chronic diseases such as ESRD, increasing activity and other lifestyle changes are difficult to implement.[11] Results of pharmacotherapy have generally been disappointing, alternating between ineffective weight loss and significant adverse effects of the medication. Some hope has been seen using high-protein diets in the general population. When used as a dietary supplement, devoid of additional fats or sugars, high-protein meals may lead to a ketosis, whereby the body's fat deposits are metabolized for energy. However, these diets may be unsafe in patients with CKD, as increased protein loads may lead to decreased kidney function and potential organ damage.[12]

The increasingly positive outcomes of bariatric surgery in the general population have led many to wonder whether bariatric surgery is appropriate in patients hoping to become eligible for transplantation. However, one major barrier to widespread implementation has been the proposed safety of surgical intervention in patients with CKD. To this end, several case reports and case series have aimed to examine the outcomes in this high-risk population.

In one such series, 3 patients with ESRD underwent laparoscopic adjustable gastric-band placement to qualify for renal transplantation. All 3 patients lost a variable amount of weight between 12 and 15 months after adjustable gastric-band placement (excess weight loss ranging from 35% to 41%), subsequently allowing for transplantation to

Table 1
Body mass index of incident patients with end-stage renal disease (ESRD) in 2010

ESRD Modality	N	Mean	SD	Median	Minimum	Maximum	Range
Hemodialysis	103,181	29.4	7.9	27.9	13.0	70.0	57.0
Peritoneal dialysis	7435	28.9	7.0	28.1	13.0	68.7	55.7
Transplantation	2424	27.4	6.3	26.8	13.0	69.4	56.4

Abbreviation: SD, standard deviation.

Data from United States Renal Data System. USRDS 2012 Annual Data Report: atlas of chronic kidney disease and end-stage renal disease in the United States. 2012. Available at: http://www.usrds.org/adr.aspx. Accessed April 4, 2013. The interpretation and reporting of these data are the responsibility of the author(s) and in no way should be seen as an official policy or interpretation of the U.S. government.

proceed.[13] The adjustable gastric band is an attractive option in that it has a very low perioperative complication rate; however, the durability of the operation is questionable because of weight regain and a high risk of long-term complications requiring removal or revision of the adjustable gastric band.[14] In this series, although the BMI criterion for transplantation was met, the follow-up was too short to assess long-term success with the band. Furthermore, 1 patient did have a substantial weight regain.

Using Medicare billing claims within the US Renal Data System registry, Modanlou and colleagues[15] described the use of open bariatric surgery in patients with renal failure, both pretransplant and posttransplant. Thirty-day mortality of wait-list patients undergoing bariatric surgery was found to be 3.5%, which is increased relative to the general population undergoing bariatric surgery. However, these cases were performed in an open fashion, contrary to the current status of bariatric surgery whereby most procedures are performed laparoscopically. The current era of laparoscopic bariatric surgery has demonstrated complication rates that are superior to those of the traditional open era. Current complication rates, taking into account both major and minor complications within 30 days of operation, have been found to be 4.3%, with 30-day mortality cited as 0.13%.[16,17] In the Modanlou study, nearly 70% of the candidates who underwent bariatric surgery while on the wait list were ultimately transplanted.

An earlier series by Alexander and colleagues[18] also examined patients undergoing gastric bypass both pretransplant and posttransplant. Nineteen patients with CKD underwent gastric bypass before renal transplantation (**Fig. 3**). At 3 years' follow-up the patients had an average excess weight loss of 79.8%, with 7 patients listed or scheduled for transplantation. By 12 months after bariatric surgery, the reduction in excess BMI was 66% and the average BMI among the group was 34.6. As expected, the patients also had significant improvements in obesity-related comorbidities such as diabetes, hypertension, and hyperlipidemia. The only perioperative complication among the group was a wound separation. No patients required blood transfusions in the perioperative period, even though nearly all the procedures were performed in an open fashion.

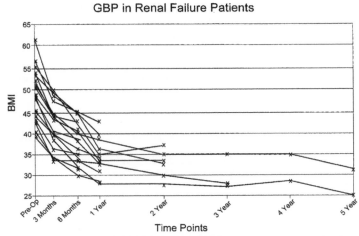

Fig. 3. Change in body mass index (BMI) of 19 patients with chronic kidney disease undergoing open gastric bypass (GBP). (*From* Alexander JW, Goodman HR, Gersin K, et al. Gastric bypass in morbidly obese patients with chronic renal failure and kidney transplant. Transplantation 2004;78(3):470; with permission.)

More recently, laparoscopic sleeve gastrectomy (LSG) has gained acceptance as an effective weight-loss procedure. Sleeve gastrectomy involves the resection of approximately two-thirds of the stomach, thereby reducing its capacity. Contrary to a Roux-en-Y gastric bypass, there is no malabsorption and no intestinal anastomoses. The decreased complexity of the operation makes it an attractive option in high-risk patients. Takata and colleagues[19] retrospectively examined their experience of laparoscopic Roux-en-Y gastric bypass (LRYGB) and LSG in ESRD patients (**Table 2**). The mean operative times to complete LSG were shorter than those for the LRYGB patients. There were no complications within the two groups. At 9 months' follow-up, excess weight loss between the two groups was equivalent, around 60% (**Fig. 4**). Although the numbers were small, the article aimed to show that sleeve gastrectomy may be an effective alternative to Roux-en-Y gastric bypass in helping morbidly obese patients become eligible for transplant.

The protocol for morbidly obese CKD and ESRD patients at the authors' institution is to proceed with an LRYGB. Of the 7 patients who have undergone bariatric surgery from 2010 to the present, there have been no perioperative complications. The surgical protocol involves dialysis the morning presurgery. Before sedation, patients receive a subcutaneous dose of enoxaparin. Postoperatively, patients are mobilized within 2 hours and undergo early feeding with clear liquids the evening of surgery. The diet is advanced to full liquids on the first postoperative day. Dialysis is performed again the morning of postoperative day 2, followed by discharge home. The average length of stay was 2.5 days. Six of these patients were on hemodialysis and 1 had grade 4 CKD. Preoperative BMI ranged from 38.7 to 56.4. All patients attained BMI eligibility for transplant within 6 months (**Table 3**). As the experience with sleeve gastrectomy grows, it may supplant Roux-en-Y gastric bypass as the procedure of choice in ESRD and CKD patients. At present, however, the durability and long-term results of sleeve gastrectomy are unknown. Roux-en-Y gastric bypass, on the other hand, has been shown to have excellent life-long results, relative risk reduction in mortality, and no effects on posttransplant dosing regimens.

Table 2
Perioperative outcomes of ESRD patients undergoing laparoscopic sleeve gastrectomy

Operative and Perioperative Outcomes	
Variable	ESRD (n = 7)
Operation	LRYGB
Operative time (min)	
Mean	189
Range	148–222
Mean estimated blood loss (mL)	64
Postoperative complications (n)	0
Length of hospitalization (d)	
Mean	3.0
Range	3–3

Abbreviation: LRYGB, laparoscopic Roux-en-Y gastric bypass.
From Takata MC, Campo GM, Ciovica R, et al. Laparoscopic bariatric surgery improves candidacy in morbidly obese patients awaiting transplantation. Surg Obes Relat Dis 2008;4(2):161; with permission.

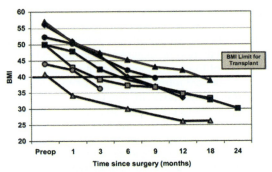

Fig. 4. Change in body mass index (BMI) in ESRD patients undergoing laparoscopic sleeve gastrectomy. (*From* Takata MC, Campo GM, Ciovica R, et al. Laparoscopic bariatric surgery improves candidacy in morbidly obese patients awaiting transplantation. Surg Obes Relat Dis 2008;4(2):163; with permission.)

RISK FACTORS FOR OBESITY IN KIDNEY TRANSPLANT RECIPIENTS

Kidney transplant recipients are at increased risk for developing or worsening obesity after transplantation. For decades it has been reported that up to 30% to 60% of kidney transplant recipients gain weight after transplantation.[1,20,21] Several factors have been identified that predispose transplant patients to an increased risk of obesity, including not only the metabolic effects imposed by posttransplant immunosuppressants but also lifestyle changes related to psychosocial factors. The most definitive study to date that evaluates the effect of corticosteroids on weight gain after transplantation established that chronic corticosteroid therapy was not the culprit in posttransplant weight gain for kidney transplant recipients.[22] On day 7 after transplantation, patients were randomized to receive either continued standard-dose corticosteroids or steroid withdrawal in a double-blind fashion. Throughout the 5-year study period after transplant, the mean weight change was not different between these 2 groups of patients.

Consequently there is also a potential need for surgical intervention in the post–kidney transplant population. Alexander and colleagues[18] detailed the outcomes of gastric bypass in 8 kidney transplant patients, whereby the pretransplant BMI of 34.3 had increased to 48.9 by the time the patients were undergoing bariatric surgery (**Fig. 5**).

Table 3			
Early results of ESRD patients undergoing laparoscopic Roux-en-Y gastric bypass at Houston Methodist Hospital's Bariatric and Metabolic Surgery Center			
Patient	Initial BMI	Time to BMI <35	Comorbidities
1	40.1	1 mo	HTN
2	48.2	6 mo	HTN
3	40.0	3 mo	DM, HTN, HLD
4	56.4	1 y	DM, HTN, OSA
5	39.9	3 mo	HTN
6	46.6		DM, HTN, HLD
7	38.7	1 mo	DM, HTN

Abbreviations: BMI, body mass index; DM, diabetes mellitus; HLD, hyperlipidemia; HTN, hypertension; OSA, obstructive sleep apnea.

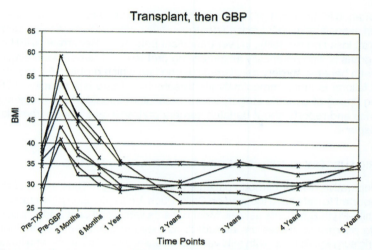

Fig. 5. Change in body mass index (BMI) in patients undergoing gastric bypass (GBP) after kidney transplant. TXP, transplantation. (*From* Alexander JW, Goodman HR, Gersin K, et al. Gastric bypass in morbidly obese patients with chronic renal failure and kidney transplant. Transplantation 2004;78(3):471; with permission.)

Along with the weight regain, patients also experienced new onset of obesity-related comorbidities such as diabetes and hypertension. Again, there were no perioperative complications or mortality in this group. Moreover, the patients did experience a significant reduction of excess BMI of 70.9%, 76.5%, and 69.7% at 1, 2, and 3 years, respectively. Considering the malabsorptive sequelae of the Roux-en-Y gastric bypass, there was a concern for altered absorption of micronutrients and immunosuppressants. Aside from steroids, however, current immunosuppressants may be effectively monitored using routine blood levels. A study of mycophenolic acid, tacrolimus, and sirolimus after gastric bypass indicated that dosing levels would likely need to be higher, to account for the differences in pharmacokinetics, than in the non-bypass population.[23]

In a separate case series, 5 renal transplant patients underwent bariatric surgery, including 4 Roux-en-Y gastric bypass and 1 sleeve gastrectomy.[24] The mean BMI was 52.2, with a range of 30 to 48. At 2 years postoperatively, patients experienced an average excess weight loss of more than 50%. The patient who underwent a sleeve gastrectomy was initially planned for a Roux-en-Y gastric bypass; however, secondary to significant intra-abdominal adhesions, the operative plan was changed to an LSG. The patient had an excellent weight loss and reduced her BMI from 48 to 31 at 2 years' follow-up. The entire group had no complications, and there were no changes reported in the dosing regimen of their immunosuppressant drugs. Although only 1 patient underwent sleeve gastrectomy, the positive results indicate the efficacy and safety of this procedure in post–kidney transplant patients.

OBESITY AND LIVER DISEASE

Obesity and liver disease are also becoming increasingly intertwined. Morbid obesity is associated with nonalcoholic fatty liver disease in 84% to 96% of patients and with nonalcoholic steatohepatitis (NASH) in 25% to 55% of patients.[25,26] With this trend in mind, several experts predict that NASH may become the most common cause of liver transplantation in the next 1 or 2 decades.[27] As with renal transplantation, obesity has also been associated with increased postoperative complications, as well as possible earlier graft loss and mortality, in liver transplant patients.[28] Recurrent NASH in transplanted grafts is also potentially an increasing problem.[29] The optimal timing of intervention with bariatric surgery may largely depend on which problem (ie, the obesity or the liver failure) is more immediately life threatening. There is a paucity of literature regarding timing of bariatric surgery in liver transplant candidates, with mostly small case series and reports about bariatric surgery pretransplant, during transplant, and posttransplant.

BARIATRIC SURGERY IN CIRRHOTIC OR PRETRANSPLANT PATIENTS

The perioperative risk for cirrhotic patients may be very high. Thus, most of the small series reported to date have focused on Child-Pugh A classification patients, with occasional Child-Pugh B patients as well. Most patients with significant portal hypertension and large perigastric varices are excluded, as they are considered contraindications to bariatric surgery. Patients with mild variceal disease, as well as some who have undergone transjugular intrahepatic portosystemic shunt (TIPS), have also been reported to have undergone bariatric surgery. In 2008, Takata and colleagues[19] published a small series of 15 morbidly obese patients who were in need of organ transplants. Six of these patients had liver disease and cirrhosis, 4 were classified as Child A, and 2 were classified as Child B. Two of the 6 developed complications, 1 of whom experienced postoperative bleeding. This patient underwent prompt reoperation, although no distinct source of bleeding was discovered. The other patient with a complication developed encephalopathy following a urinary tract infection. Mean follow-up was 9 months and there was no incidence of liver decompensation. Five of the 6 patients subsequently became candidates for liver transplantation.

The same group recently presented an abstract at the 2012 American Society of Metabolic and Bariatric Surgery annual meeting, reporting 26 pretransplant patients undergoing a sleeve gastrectomy, 20 of whom had liver disease.[30] There was 1 staple-line leak, 1 transient encephalopathy, and 1 bleed requiring a transfusion, but no mortality. Furthermore, patients experienced an excess weight loss of 50% at 12 months.

Another recent series published by Shimizu and colleagues[26] included 23 patients (22 with Child-Pugh class A and 1 with Child-Pugh class B). Fourteen patients underwent a Roux-en-Y gastric bypass, 8 patients an LSG, and 1 patient a laparoscopic adjustable gastric band. Two patients had a successful LSG after TIPS. There was no perioperative mortality, no liver decompensation, and 1 leak each in the gastric bypass and sleeve gastrectomy groups. There was an excellent mean excess weight loss of approximately 67% at 12 months' follow up. The investigators concluded that although complications are likely to be higher in this high-risk group, they do not appear to be prohibitive based on their outcomes.

An earlier series from 2004 from Dallal and colleagues[31] included 30 patients, 90% of whom were diagnosed intraoperatively as cirrhotic based on gross liver appearance. All cirrhotics were compensated, defined as absence of ascites, normal bilirubin, normal synthetic function, and no obvious portal hypertension. Twenty-seven patients underwent a Roux-en-Y gastric bypass and 3 patients underwent an LSG, 1 of which was converted to a gastric bypass as part of a staged procedure. No patient experienced liver decompensation, although there was 1 anastomotic leak. Two other complications included the need for blood transfusions and transient renal dysfunction. This series also demonstrated that although patients with compensated liver disease had a higher risk of complications, bariatric surgery could still be performed with acceptable morbidity.

BARIATRIC SURGERY DURING LIVER TRANSPLANT

In advanced liver disease, concerns regarding portal hypertension, such as bleeding, precipitating more severe hepatic dysfunction, and death, have led some to investigate the possibility of performing bariatric procedures at the time of the liver transplant. The theoretical advantage is that the portal system is decompressed, and the abdomen is already accessible to adding a procedure such as an adjustable gastric band or sleeve gastrectomy. The added time to complete the bariatric procedure would therefore be minimal. This approach also avoids the need for a repeat operation after a large open procedure when significant adhesions could potentially be encountered. Campsen and colleagues[32] reported a case of placement of an adjustable gastric band performed at the time of liver transplantation in a morbidly obese patient with hypertension, diabetes, sleep apnea, and venous stasis. The patient did well postoperatively and lost approximately 45% of excess weight by 6 months, with her BMI falling from 42 to 34. Operative time was extended by only 30 minutes.

In a recent series from the Mayo Clinic published in 2012,[29] a total of 7 patients underwent a liver transplant combined with sleeve gastrectomy. The decision to perform sleeve gastrectomy rather than a gastric bypass was attributable to the absence of malabsorption that accompanies the sleeve gastrectomy. Because gastrointestinal continuity is not affected, there would be no impact on absorption of immunosuppression drugs. Moreover, endoscopic access to the biliary tree would be preserved after the transplant. Concurrent placement of an adjustable gastric band was not performed, owing to its lesser efficacy in comparison with sleeve gastrectomy. There were no mortalities in this series, and allograft function was preserved without incident. The mean BMI was 48 at transplant and 29 postoperatively at the last follow-up. None of the patients had steatosis on follow-up, based on annual protocol ultrasonography. One patient developed a gastric staple-line leak and required multiple operations with early graft dysfunction, but eventually recovered and was able to be discharged home. There was excessive weight loss down to a BMI of 20 in 1 patient, and another required thymoglobulin for rejection, but all were found to have normal allograft function on routine follow-up. All patients received standard posttransplant immunosuppression and experienced no difficulty with tacrolimus dosing.

BARIATRIC SURGERY AFTER LIVER TRANSPLANT

Similar to the literature regarding kidney transplant patients, there is a paucity of data regarding bariatric surgery after liver transplant, except for a few case reports and small series of patients. A report published by Duchini and Brunson[33] in 2001 described 2 patients undergoing an open Roux-en-Y gastric bypass for recurrent steatohepatitis after liver transplant. Both patients had a BMI higher than 60. Their postoperative recovery was unremarkable as they did not have any significant complications. Both experienced resolution of steatohepatitis and did not require changes in tacrolimus or immunosuppression dosing.

Another case report from Tichansky and Madan[34] in 2005 described the first LRYGB in a post–liver transplant patient whose BMI was 54. This patient also had an uneventful postoperative course as well as good early weight loss. In 2007, a case report was published about a sleeve gastrectomy in a patient with an initial BMI of 47.[35] This patient had initially undergone an intragastric balloon placement to lose weight before the liver transplant. He subsequently developed a biliary stricture that required a revision to a Roux-en-Y biliary bypass. Incidentally, he had regained weight and now had a BMI of 37.9. He underwent a simultaneous open biliary bypass and a sleeve gastrectomy. Postoperatively, his BMI decreased to 29.8 at 6 months' follow-up. Moreover, his trough cyclosporine levels were stable postoperatively.

A larger recent series by Lin and colleagues[36] described sleeve gastrectomies in 9 patients with prior liver transplantation. Their choice of sleeve gastrectomy over gastric banding was made to avoid foreign-body implantation. Gastric bypass was not chosen, as they wished to maintain endoscopic biliary access and reduce the complexity of the surgical weight-loss procedure. Unfortunately, in this study there were 3 complications. One patient developed a bile leak from the liver surface, which subsequently resolved with drainage and argon-beam coagulation. Another patient had a simultaneous repair of a large incisional hernia and experienced a dehiscence on postoperative day 2, the treatment of which required a reoperation. The third patient developed persistent dysphagia. Manometry was performed, which demonstrated aperistalsis of the esophagus, despite no significant anatomic deformities or mechanical obstructions seen during upper endoscopy. The patient underwent a subsequent revision to a Roux-en-Y gastric bypass, whereby the symptoms resolved. Weight loss was significant, with the patient reaching 55.5% of excess weight loss at 6 months. Calcineurin-inhibitor levels remained stable.

SUMMARY

As the incidence of obesity continues to increase, so too do obesity-related comorbidities. The number of patients with morbid obesity who also presenting with end-stage organ dysfunction is also increasing. The increased incidence of hypertension and diabetes has led to an increase in incidence of CKD, and the prevalence of metabolic syndrome and NASH has also led to increased numbers of cirrhotic patients. Morbid obesity is a barrier to transplantation, as these patients have been found to have increased risk of complications and allograft loss. Weight loss is necessary not only to help patients become eligible for transplantation based on BMI criteria but also to help improve or resolve obesity-related comorbidities, which independently increase the risk of mortality.

Unfortunately, there are few data to guide physicians and surgeons regarding the optimal intervention or the timing of such intervention. In the case of patients with CKD and dialysis, bariatric surgery has been shown to be safe and effective, even in the setting of ESRD. Regarding patients with cirrhosis and liver failure, it appears that the best time to intervene is before significant portal hypertension or liver synthetic dysfunction has occurred. Physicians caring for these patients must therefore be more aggressive with weight management in the early stages of liver disease, especially with patients with NASH who have not yet developed portal hypertension. Once patients develop portal hypertension and varices, surgical weight loss may become prohibitive. However, in patients with a high risk of perioperative complications and mortality, procedures such as sleeve gastrectomy may provide a less complicated operation than a Roux-en-Y gastric bypass, with similar efficacy for weight loss. Furthermore, endoscopic surveillance of the biliary tree is maintained in a sleeve gastrectomy. However, in patients with gastric varices, division of the short gastric vessels, which is necessary to remove the fundus in a sleeve gastrectomy, may lead to redirection of blood elsewhere and subsequent worsening of the portal hypertension, in addition to the significant risk of bleeding from the divided vessels. However, there is some precedent set with devascularization procedures of the stomach, which have been used with limited success for severe variceal bleeding. Creation of the pouch in a gastric bypass obviates the division of any vasculature along the greater curvature; however, the procedure results in an inability to endoscopically survey the bypassed stomach where gastric varices may lead to a life-threatening bleed. Obviously there are many factors in morbidly obese patients with liver disease to be considered when attempting to ensure the safety of any bariatric procedure.

Clinical course will dictate timing as well. Patients with ESRD may survive for prolonged periods on hemodialysis, thereby enlarging the window for intervention. However, in patients with morbid obesity, severe liver disease, and portal hypertension, therapeutic options may be limited. In these patients, intervention with TIPS may help decrease portal hypertension, which may then decrease the perioperative risk for bariatric surgery. If bariatric surgery is not performed before synthetic dysfunction and portal hypertension are present, and the patients still qualify for liver transplant, it may be prudent to wait until after recovery from transplantation to intervene.

REFERENCES

1. Glanton C, Kao T, Cruess D, et al. Impact of renal transplantation on survival in end-stage renal disease patients with elevated body mass index. Kidney Int 2003;63(2):647–53.
2. Bunnapradist S, Danovitch G. Evaluation of adult kidney transplant candidates. Am J Kidney Dis 2007;50(5):890–8.
3. Knoll G, Cockfield S, Blydt-Hansen T, et al. Canadian Society of Transplantation consensus guidelines on eligibility for kidney transplantation. Can Med Assoc J 2007;173(10):S1–25.
4. Meier-Kriesche H, Amdorfer J, Kaplan B. The impact of body mass index on renal transplant outcomes: a significant independent risk factor for graft failure and patient death. Transplantation 2002;73(1):70–4.
5. Byers T. Body weight and mortality. N Engl J Med 1995;333:723–4.
6. Mokdad A, Serdula MK, Dietz WH, et al. The spread of the obesity epidemic in the United States, 1991-1998. JAMA 1999;282(16):1519–22.
7. Flegal K, Kit B, Orpana H, et al. Association of all-cause mortality with overweight and obesity using standard body mass index categories: a systematic review and meta-analysis. J Am Med Assn 2013;309(1):72–82.
8. U.S. Renal Data System. USRDS 2012 annual data report: atlas of chronic kidney disease and end-stage renal disease in the United States. 2012. Available at: http://www.usrds.org/adr.aspx. Accessed April 4, 2013.
9. Eckel RH. Nonsurgical management of obesity in adults. N Engl J Med 2008;358: 1941–50.
10. Council on Scientific Affairs. Treatment of obesity in adults. JAMA 1988;260: 2547–51.
11. Teta D. Weight loss in obese patients with chronic kidney disease: who and how? J Ren Care 2010;36(Suppl 1):163–71.
12. Cano NJ, Aparicio M, Brunori G, et al, ESPEN. ESPEN Guidelines on parenteral nutrition: adult renal failure. Clin Nutr 2009;28:401–4.
13. Koshy AN, Coombes JS,.Wilkinson S, et al. Laparoscopic gastric banding surgery performed in obese dialysis patients prior to kidney transplantation. Am J Kidney Dis 2008;52(4):e15–7.
14. Himpens J, Cadiere GB, Bazi M, et al. Long-term outcomes of laparoscopic adjustable gastric banding. Arch Surg 2011;146(7):802–7.

15. Modanlou KA, Mithyala U, Xiao H, et al. Bariatric surgery among kidney transplant candidates and recipients: analysis of the United States Renal Data System and literature review. Transplantation 2009;87(8):1167–73.
16. The Longitudinal Assessment of Bariatric Surgery (LABS) Consortium. Perioperative safety in the longitudinal assessment of bariatric surgery. N Engl J Med 2009;361:445–54.
17. DeMaria EJ, Pate V, Warthen M, et al. Baseline data from American Society for Metabolic and Bariatric Surgery-designated bariatric surgery centers of excellence using the bariatric outcomes longitudinal database. Surg Obes Relat Dis 2010;6:347–55.
18. Alexander JW, Goodman HR, Gersin K, et al. Gastric bypass in morbidly obese patients with chronic renal failure and kidney transplant. Transplantation 2004; 78(3):469–74.
19. Takata MC, Campo GM, Ciovica R, et al. Laparoscopic bariatric surgery improves candidacy in morbidly obese patients awaiting transplantation. Surg Obes Relat Dis 2008;4(2):159–64.
20. Moore L, Gaber AO. Patterns of early weight change after renal transplantation. J Ren Nutr 1996;6:21–5.
21. Pischon T, Sharma AM. Obesity as a risk factor in renal transplant patients. Nephrol Dial Transplant 2001;16(1):14–7.
22. Woodle ES, First MR, Pirsch J, et al. A prospective, randomized, double-blind, placebo-controlled multicenter trial comparing early (7 day) corticosteroid cessation versus long-term, low-dose corticosteroid therapy. Ann Surg 2008;248(4): 564–77.
23. Rogers CC, Alloway RR, Alexander JW, et al. Pharmacokinetics of mycophenolic acid, tacrolimus and sirolimus after gastric bypass surgery in end-stage renal disease and transplant patients: a pilot study. Clin Transplant 2008;22:281–91.
24. Szomstein S, Rojas R, Rosenthal RJ. Outcomes of laparoscopic bariatric surgery after renal transplant. Obes Surg 2010;20:383–5.
25. Gholam PM, Kotler DP, Flancbaum LJ. Liver pathology in morbidly obese patients undergoing Roux-en-Y gastric bypass surgery. Obes Surg 2002;12:49–51.
26. Shimizu H, Phuong V, Maia A, et al. Bariatric surgery in patients with liver cirrhosis. Surg Obes Relat Dis 2013;9(1):1–6.
27. Mandell MS, Zimmerman M, Campsen J, et al. Bariatric surgery in liver transplant patients: weighing the evidence. Obes Surg 2008;18:1515–6.
28. Nair S, Verma S, Thuluvath PJ. Obesity and its effect on survival in patients undergoing orthotopic liver transplantation in the United States. Hepatology 2002;35: 105–9.
29. Heimbach JK, Watt KD, Poterucha JJ, et al. Combined liver transplantation and gastric sleeve resection for patients with medically complicated obesity and end-stage liver disease. Am J Transplant 2013;13(2):363–8.
30. Lin MY, Sarin A, Tavakoll M, et al. Laparoscopic sleeve gastrectomy is safe and efficacious for pretransplant candidates. Abstract PL-117, from 2012 ASMBS Annual Meeting.
31. Dallal RM, Mattar SG, Lord JL, et al. Results of laparoscopic gastric bypass in patients with cirrhosis. Obes Surg 2004;14:47–53.
32. Campsen JZ, Shoen J, Wachs M, et al. Adjustable gastric banding in a morbidly obese patient during liver transplantation. Obes Surg 2008;18:1625–7.
33. Duchini A, Brunson ME. Roux-en Y gastric bypass for recurrent nonalcoholic steatohepatitis in liver transplant recipients with morbid obesity. Transplantation 2001;72:156–9.

34. Tichansky DS, Madan AK. Laparoscopic Roux-en-Y gastric bypass is safe and feasible after orthotopic liver transplantation. Obes Surg 2005;15:1481–6.
35. Butte JM, Devaud N, Jarufe N, et al. Sleeve gastrectomy as treatment for severe obesity after orthotopic liver transplantation. Obes Surg 2007;17(11):1517–9.
36. Lin MY, Tavakol MM, Sarin A, et al. Safety and feasibility of sleeve gastrectomy in morbidly obese patients following liver transplantation. Surg Endosc 2013; 27:81–5.

Advances in Lung Preservation

Tiago N. Machuca, MD, PhD, Marcelo Cypel, MD, MSc,
Shaf Keshavjee, MD, MSc*

KEYWORDS

- Lung transplantation • Organ preservation • Ex vivo lung perfusion
- Organ procurement • Non–heart beating donor

KEY POINTS

- Conventional lung preservation is centered on cold ischemia in order to slow cell metabolism and prevent organ deterioration.
- Ex vivo lung perfusion (EVLP) has emerged as a modern technique that preserves lungs on a functional state using protective perfusion/ventilation strategies.
- EVLP has been successfully translated to clinical practice; donor lungs deemed unsuitable for transplantation underwent EVLP and were ultimately transplanted, rendering similar outcomes as those from conventional donor lungs.
- Because it can safely preserve donor lungs for extended periods in a metabolically active state, EVLP provides the ideal platform for repeated lung evaluation, allowing the employment of diagnostic tools to guide the delivery of injury-specific therapies.

LUNG SHORTAGE AND POTENTIAL ALTERNATIVES TO EXPAND THE DONOR POOL

Lung transplantation is a well-established therapy for patients with end-stage lung disease. The 2012 report from the International Society for Heart and Lung Transplantation Registry has shown that since the mid 90s, there has been a steady increase in the number of procedures performed yearly, with a peak of 3519 cases in its most recent year, 2010.[1] However, although lung transplant activity clearly increased, the number of patients being listed has increased in proportions that are much higher.[2] Because the number of donor lungs suitable for transplantation cannot fulfill the requirements of the growing demand, the mortality while waiting for a lung is still considerable. In the United States, despite the initial decrease after implementation of the Lung Allocation

Disclosures: S. Keshavjee and M. Cypel were principal investigators for the Toronto Ex-Vivo Lung Perfusion Trial sponsored by Vitrolife, a company that makes sterile solutions for organ preservation.
S. Keshavjee and M. Cypel are founding members of Perfusix Inc, a company that provides ex-vivo organ perfusion services.
Toronto Lung Transplant Program, Toronto General Hospital, University Health Network, University of Toronto, 200 Elizabeth Street, 9N969, Toronto, Ontario M5G 2C4, Canada
* Corresponding author.
E-mail address: shaf.keshavjee@uhn.ca

Surg Clin N Am 93 (2013) 1373–1394
http://dx.doi.org/10.1016/j.suc.2013.08.001
0039-6109/13/$ – see front matter © 2013 Elsevier Inc. All rights reserved.
surgical.theclinics.com

Score (LAS), the wait-list mortality has increased again.[2] Furthermore, in a national study reporting the UK experience, the wait-list mortality was 35%, approaching close to 50% for indications such as bronchiectasis and interstitial lung disease.[3]

Although other organs are protected from the external environment, the lung is prone to a series of injuries during the donation process (such as ventilator-acquired pneumonia, neurogenic and hydrostatic pulmonary edema, barotrauma), rendering very low utilization rates. In the United States, only 17.3% of lungs were recovered from organ donors by 2008. In that same year, 6578 consented organ donors did not undergo lung procurement because of poor organ function.[4]

Potential ways to address this issue have been previously explored. Although the use of donors that do not fulfill the conventional lung donation criteria has been previously reported as successful in smaller series, larger cohorts have shown a higher incidence of primary graft dysfunction (PGD) (43.9% vs 27.4% in Botha and colleagues)[5] and higher 30-day mortality (17.5% vs 6.2% in Pierre and colleagues).[6]

Since its successful initial report,[7] the use of donors after cardiac death (DCD) has been explored as a valuable source of lungs. In the setting of controlled cardiac death (Maastricht category III, donors awaiting cardiac arrest), series of reports have described the increasing international experience.[8–12] Although excellent outcomes can be achieved, as depicted by the report of Levvey and colleagues[13] with 1-year survival of 97%, results inferior to those of brain death donors have also been described.[14] The potential injuries that the lung may suffer after extubation (hypoxia and aspiration) and during the agonal phase (prolonged hypotension, warm ischemia) are likely responsible for these inferior results and may also explain the caution generally observed in the transplant community whenever considering donation after cardiac death.

Focusing on the expansion of the donor pool, some pioneer groups have moved further on the use of donors after uncontrolled cardiac death (Maastricht categories I and II). Although supported as an alternative to death on the wait list, higher rates of PGD grade 2 to 3 were reported (53%), with a 1-year survival of 69%.[15]

Another option, already currently used by a large number of lung transplant programs, has been recently highlighted. Data from 1295 transplants reported by the UK Registry have shown how the use of lungs from donors with a smoking history provides a net benefit to patients on the wait list. Nevertheless, this initial advantage came at a cost of worse long-term outcomes when compared with recipients of lungs from nonsmokers.[16]

Based on all of these specific issues related to organ donation, ex vivo lung perfusion (EVLP) has emerged as a promising preservation technique to increase the utilization rate and provide safe lungs that would otherwise be discarded, rendering similar outcomes as those obtained with donors accepted under conventional criteria.[17]

After a brief review of conventional lung preservation, this article discusses the rationale behind EVLP and how it has shifted the paradigm of organ preservation from conventional static cold ischemia to the utilization of functional normothermia, restoring the lung's own metabolism and its reparative processes. Technical aspects and previous clinical experience as well as opportunities to address specific donor organ injuries in a personalized medicine approach are also reviewed.

CONVENTIONAL LUNG PRESERVATION

For years, donor lung preservation was centered on cold static preservation, a process that aims to slow cell metabolism and reduce oxygen and other substrate requirements, ultimately preventing organ deterioration. Because most of the detrimental effects of hypoxia/ischemia are driven by chemical reactions, it seems logical to reduce the organ temperature in order to reduce enzymatic activity related to these processes. However, because this strategy is nonselective, vital enzymes, such as Na^+-K^+ ATPase, have also decreased function, causing an ionic imbalance that leads to cell edema and injury.[18] Besides, intracellular calcium accumulation causes further cell damage and, although the lung benefits from inflation with oxygen, it has been shown that the generation of reactive oxygen species also occurs during cold ischemia.[19,20]

Experimental work showed that, as opposed to kidney and liver, lung preservation was significantly superior when the flushing solution had extracellular characteristics.[21,22] Moreover, the specific contributions of a low potassium concentration and dextran 40 on the quality of preservation were further ellucidated.[23] With regard to the volume of flush, it has been shown that 60 mL/kg results in effective flush cooling, more homogeneous flush, and improved lung function when compared with 20 mL/kg.[24]

The optimal solution temperature has been investigated; although studies with small animals have shown the benefits of using solutions at 23°C[25] or 15°C to 20°C[26] instead of 10°C, it has been generally accepted that in the clinical scenario, lower temperatures are required to achieve similar core organ temperatures. It has also been reported that the storage of lungs at 10°C yields superior results than at 4°C.[27] Nevertheless, for both flush solution and organ storage in the clinical setting, the impracticality of using tightly temperature-controlled containers added to the deleterious effect of using higher temperatures with narrower safety margins has supported the routine use of the 4°C to 8°C range.

One key aspect in which lungs have an advantage over other organs is the ability to preserve them inflated with oxygen, thus allowing for ongoing energy-efficient aerobic metabolism. The benefits of this strategy in maintaining the integrity of the alveolocapillary barrier have been shown.[28,29]

The theoretical advantages of a retrograde flush in clearing blood from the bronchial circulation and also in removing potential clots from the pulmonary circulation, ultimately leading to a better flushing, have been demonstrated experimentally and widely adopted clinically.[30]

The conventional lung preservation method is only briefly reviewed here because extensive reviews have been reported elsewhere.[31,32] **Table 1** depicts the current protocol from the Toronto Lung Transplant Program for cold static preservation; as one can see, there have been no major changes over the last 2 decades.

EVLP

With all the aforementioned measures, clinical lung transplantation has largely evolved since the 80s, gaining worldwide acceptance and rendering better outcomes. However, candidates are still dying on the wait list, and recipients are still presenting with PGD. The search for better preservation techniques to not only safely expand the pool of donors but to also provide better, more reliable organs led to the development of EVLP.

The idea of perfusing whole organs outside the body is not new. In fact, using a sterile chamber, Alexis Carrel and Charles Lindbergh[33] were able to perfuse whole organs, such as thyroid, ovary, adrenal glands, spleen, heart, and kidney, as early as 1935. From the 60s to the 90s, research in EVLP was mainly regarded as a method to study pulmonary physiology. It was in 2000 that Steen first translated the EVLP application

Table 1
Conventional static lung preservation technique (Toronto Lung Transplant Program)

Preservation Solution	Perfadex
Pharmacologic manipulation	500 mcg PGE_1 into the PA before cross-clamp and in the flush solution
Volume antegrade flush	60 mL/kg
Volume of retrograde flush	250 mL/pulmonary vein
PA pressure during flush	10–15 mm Hg (30 cm height above donor heart)
Temperature of flush solution	4°C–8°C
Lung ventilation during flush	V_T: 10 mL/kg, PEEP 5 cm H_2O
Oxygenation	$F_{IO_2} = 50\%$
Lung inflation during storage	15–20 cm H_2O
Storage temperature	4°C–8°C

Abbreviations: PGE_1, prostaglandin E1; V_T, tidal volume.
Modified from de Perrot M, Keshavjee S. Lung preservation. Semin Thorac Cardiovasc Surg 2004;16:300–8.

to organ evaluation. Aiming for a short period of assessment of lungs from donors after cardiac arrest, he successfully established a technique using an extracellular colloid solution based on human albumin and dextran. The Toronto group further developed the concept of extended EVLP, focusing on providing a platform not only for repeated periodic reassessment but also to allow organ treatment in the normothermic state.[34,35]

Isolated human lung perfusion experiments from Matthay's laboratory have previously shown the beneficial effect of pulmonary vascular perfusion on alveolar fluid clearance.[36] Using lungs from the same donor, alveolar fluid clearance was more than 4 times higher in lungs that were normothermically perfused as compared with those submitted to passive rewarming. Furthermore, experiments with human lungs resected because of lung cancer have shown the absence of alveolar fluid clearance under hypothermic conditions.[37] Although pulmonary perfusion is beneficial, one should note that EVLP with high flows translates into worsened histology, weight gain, and ultimately impaired pulmonary physiology.[38–40] To avoid the deleterious hemodynamic stresses elicited by reperfusion of a previously hypothermic organ, the authors' strategy advocates low, protective flows that are gradually increased during lung rewarming.[41–43] The authors' target flow consists of 40% of the predicted donor cardiac output.

Broccard and coworkers[44] studied the role of positive atrial pressure in an isolated lung perfusion model. Using rabbit lungs, they reported that under the same vascular flow and the same ventilation protocol, experiments that maintained an atrial pressure of 6 cm H_2O developed less edema formation and lower ultrafiltration coefficients. More importantly, they reported vascular failure (pulmonary hypertension, accelerated weight gain, and capillary leakage) in all but one case in the group with an atrial pressure of 1 mm Hg as opposed to none in the cases with an atrial pressure of 6 mm Hg.[44] In a similar study using rat lungs, Petak and coworkers[45] have shown that atrial pressure plays an important role on pulmonary mechanical properties. Their results suggested that atrial pressures that are either more than or less than the physiologic range may be detrimental.[45]

The perfusate used during EVLP, Steen solution (XVIVO, Vitrolife, Englewood, CO, USA), is an extracellular solution with the addition of human albumin and dextran 40.

Albumin is instrumental in maintaining optimal colloid osmotic pressure. It has been shown to prevent edema formation in models of lung perfusion.[46,47] Dextran is known to protect the endothelium from complement injury and cell-mediated cytotoxicity and also inhibits both coagulation cascade and platelet aggregation.[48,49] Furthermore, the positive effects of dextran on lung preservation have been previously demonstrated.[23,50] Although some groups have added red blood cells to Steen solution as their perfusate, there are no data suggesting additional lung preservation advantages with this strategy. The authors have found the addition of red cells to be prohibitive in extended normothermic EVLP using the currently available perfusion technology.

The rationale behind the mechanical ventilation strategy adopted in EVLP comes from evidence of randomized clinical trials in patients with acute lung injury/acute respiratory distress syndrome pointing to significantly better outcomes, expressed as a lower mortality rate and less days on the ventilator, in patients ventilated with lower (6 mL/kg) as opposed to higher tidal volumes (12 mL/kg).[51,52] The use of similar protective ventilation after allograft reperfusion has been shown to improve lung injury histologically and decrease levels of proinflammatory cytokines, leading to better pulmonary function.[53]

CURRENT EVLP TECHNIQUE AT TORONTO GENERAL HOSPITAL

After the standard donor assessment, lungs deemed high risk for clinical transplantation are assigned to EVLP. The current indications for EVLP are listed in **Box 1**.

Lung procurement follows conventional technique. However, a few details deserve mention when considering EVLP. When the heart is being simultaneously recovered, one can expect shorter left atrial and pulmonary artery (PA) cuffs; this is not a particular problem for EVLP preparation. Very short atrial cuffs can be sutured to the cannula; at the time of cannula removal, the running Prolene (Ethicon Inc, Somerville, NJ) suture is simply cut and no length of atrial cuff tissue is lost. Furthermore, in cases when the main PA has been cut very short, at its bifurcation, it can be sewn to the specifically designed PA cannula. With respect to the airway, in the conventional lung donor procedure, the procurement team should be aware of the requirement of a longer portion of the trachea to have sufficient trachea to intubate during EVLP; hence, the donor trachea should be stapled across just below the larynx.

Box 1
Current indications for EVLP for both brain death donors and donors after cardiac death

1. Best Pao_2/Fio_2 less than 300 mm Hg

2. Signs of pulmonary edema either on chest radiograph or physical examination at the donor site

3. Poor lung compliance during examination at procurement operation

4. High-risk history, such as more than 10 units of blood transfusion or questionable history of aspiration

5. DCDs with more than 60-minute interval from withdrawal life support to cardiac arrest

Modified from Cypel M, Yeung JC, Liu M, et al. Normothermic ex vivo lung perfusion in clinical lung transplantation. N Engl J Med 2011;364:1431–40; and Cypel M, Yeung JC, Machuca T, et al. Experience with the first 50 ex vivo lung perfusions in clinical transplantation. J Thorac Cardiovasc Surg 2012;144:1200–6.

After arrival at the transplant center, the lungs are prepared on the back table. Careful re-inspection for macroscopic focal or generalized abnormalities should be done at this moment. The vascular structures are revised. After this step, the left atrium (LA) is prepared for the suture of a dedicated atrial cannula (made of stiffer plastic to favor drainage of the pulmonary veins). The authors use running sutures with 4-0 Prolene (**Fig. 1**). Next, the PA cannula is inserted into the main PA and tied with 2 heavy silk ties. If the PA is too short for cannula insertion, a dedicated cuffed PA cannula can then be trimmed to size and similarly sutured with a running 5-0 Prolene suture (**Fig. 2**). The trachea is then dissected, opened below the stapler line, and intubated with a conventional endotracheal tube. The use of a clamp above the carina prevents lung deflation during this step. The endotracheal tube is then secured with 2 heavy silk ties (**Fig. 3**). The endotracheal tube is clamped, and the carinal clamp is removed. At this moment, the still-inflated lung has been intubated and connected with the PA and LA cannulae, ready to be placed on the EVLP system. The final appearance of the lungs after cannulation is depicted in **Fig. 4**A. A second retrograde flush with 1 L of Perfadex (Vitrolife, Englewood, CO, USA) is now performed. One often sees blood clots and fat emboli in the effluent. The LA and PA cannulation connections are checked for leaks at this time, and any leaks are sutured securely to essentially create a watertight lung perfusion system.

Single-Lung EVLP

Technical aspects for single-lung EVLP include the possibility of ventilating the right lung through the trachea, with the left stump amputated at its takeoff (**Fig. 5**). For single-left lung perfusions, because the left main bronchus is longer than the right, intubation can be easily performed through it. Both right and left main PAs are usually long enough to allow separate cannulation. However, ligation of the contralateral PA allows simpler cannulation of the main PA. Nevertheless, it is possible to perfuse donor lungs simultaneously as 2 separate single lungs. The authors have adopted this strategy whenever one lung is considered for clinical EVLP and the contralateral one is deemed too damaged and allocated for EVLP at the research laboratory.

The EVLP Circuit

The authors currently use a dedicated circuit for EVLP (**Fig. 6**). It is composed of a centrifugal pump, a leukocyte filter, a hollow-fiber oxygenator heat exchanger, and a hard-shell reservoir, all connected with three-eighths tubing. After circuit assembly, it is

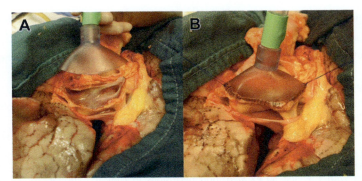

Fig. 1. Attachment of the left atrial cannula. (*A*) 2 edge sutures are placed in the atrial cuff (no simultaneous heart procurement), (*B*) final aspect of the atrial cuff - cannula running suture.

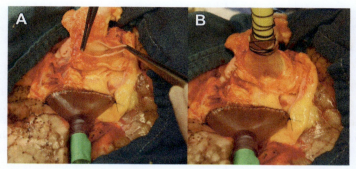

Fig. 2. Insertion and securing of the PA cannula. (*A*) Same case depicted in **Fig. 1**, with a long main PA, (*B*) PA cannula is inserted and secured with heavy silk ties.

primed with 2.0 L of Steen solution, 500 mg methylprednisolone (Solu-Medrol, Sandoz Canada, Boucherville, Canada), 3000 IU of unfractionated heparin (Organon, Canada), and antibiotic (500 mg imipenem/cilastatin, Primaxin, Merck, Whitehouse Station, NJ). In cases of excessive leak through either the LA or PA sutures, a roller pump can be added to the circuit to facilitate recirculation of the leaked fluid. However, every attempt should be made to repair any leaks to keep the circuit closed as much as possible.

Initiation and Steady State

The lungs are placed in the EVLP chamber. A cotton lap sponge placed beneath the lung prevents excessive sliding or displacement in the chamber once ventilation starts. Antegrade perfusion is started; once the PA cannula is completely filled with Steen solution, it is connected to the circuit (see **Fig. 4**B). Once the LA cannula is filled with Steen solution, it is connected to the circuit, de-airing as much as possible. The outflow clamp is then removed, and perfusion is initiated with 10% of the previously calculated target flow (see **Fig. 4**C). At 10 minutes, the set temperature of the heater-cooler is increased to 30°C and flow is increased to 20%. At any incremental flow change, the LA pressure is carefully checked and reset if necessary to be maintained between 3 and 5 mm Hg by adjusting the height of the reservoir. At 20 minutes, the temperature is increased to 37°C in the heater-cooler and flow is increased to 30%

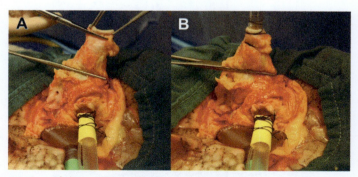

Fig. 3. Preparation of the trachea. (*A*) Clamp is placed above the carina to keep the lungs inflated and the trachea is opened just below the staple line. (*B*) A conventional endotracheal tube is inserted and secured with heavy silk ties.

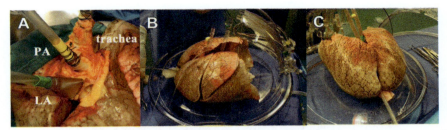

Fig. 4. (*A*) Final view of the lungs after cannulation. (*B*) Lungs placed in EVLP chamber, ready to start priming. (*C*) Initiation of perfusion.

of calculated full flow. When the system reaches 32°C, ventilation is initiated with 7 mL/kg, positive end-expiratory pressure (PEEP) of 5 cm H_2O, and 7 cycles per minute. On ventilation, the gas mixture (86% N_2, 8% CO_2, and 6% O_2) should be turned on at a sweep of 1 L/min. The sweep should be titrated to maintain a postmembrane Pco_2 between 35 and 40 mm Hg. At 30, 40, and 50 minutes, the flow will be increased to 50%, 80%, and 100% of the target, respectively. Once the lung is normothermic, perfused with target flow and ventilated, alveolar recruitment maneuvers up to 25 cm H_2O are performed. The lung has now reached the steady state (see **Fig. 6**). The LA pressure tends to be more stable from this point on, rarely requiring additional adjustments of the reservoir level. At the first hour, the authors exchange 500 mL of Steen solution from the circuit and then 250 mL hourly thereafter. Recruitment maneuvers are performed 30 minutes after each assessment.

Assessment Mode

At each hour, ventilation parameters are changed to 10 mL/kg tidal volume, 10 beats per minute (bpm), and a fraction of inspired oxygen (Fio_2) of 1.0 for 5 minutes; perfusate samples from the venous and arterial side are collected for gas analysis (**Fig. 7**). Assessment also includes PA pressure, LA pressure, peak airway pressure, plateau pressure, and dynamic and static compliance. A lung radiograph is routinely performed at 1 hour and then every 2 hours thereafter. Criteria for lung acceptance or declination for transplantation after EVLP are depicted in **Box 2**. The authors have described the impact of an acellular perfusate on EVLP assessment. With careful

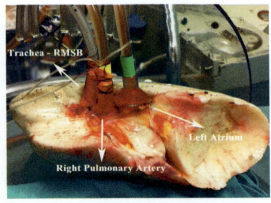

Fig. 5. View of adapted cannulation technique for single-lung perfusion (right lung). RMSB, right main stem bronchus.

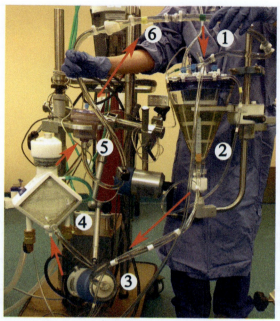

Fig. 6. The Toronto EVLP circuit. Circuit is primed with 2 L of Steen solution, heparin, methylprednisolone, and imipenem. (1) Outflow end (*green*), which will be connected to the atrial cannula; (2) hard-shell reservoir; (3) centrifugal pump; (4) heater/cooler and gas exchange membrane; (5) leukocyte filter; (6) inflow end (*yellow*), which will be connected to the pulmonary artery cannula. Red arrows denote the direction of flow.

analysis, they have demonstrated that ventilation physiology and pulmonary mechanics (peak airway pressure, compliance) are more sensitive markers of donor lung quality than the perfusate Po_2, which hitherto was viewed as the gold standard for donor lung assessment, in vivo. Trends of worsening peak airway pressure and compliance will become evident before deterioration in oxygenation performance of the ex vivo perfused lung.[54] Therefore, these parameters should be observed carefully.

Termination of Perfusion

The authors usually make a decision on acceptability of the lung at 3 hours of EVLP. Their protocol encompasses perfusion for at least 4 hours. If at this time it is not

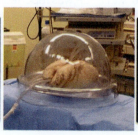

Steady State	Assessment
•Tidal volume 7 mL/kg	•Tidal volume 10 mL/kg
•Rate 7 cycles/min	•Rate 10 cycles/min
•FIO$_2$ 21%	•FIO$_2$ 100%
•PEEP 5 cm H$_2$O	•PEEP 5 cm H$_2$O

Fig. 7. EVLP: steady state and assessment mode ventilation settings.

Box 2
Acceptance and exclusion criteria after 4 to 6 hours of clinical EVLP

Acceptance criteria after EVLP

1. Pao_2/Fio_2 ratio more than 400 mm Hg

2. Stable or improving pulmonary artery pressure

3. Stable or improving airway pressure

4. Stable or improving pulmonary compliance

Exclusion criteria after EVLP

1. Pao_2/Fio_2 ratio less than 400 mm Hg

2. Greater than 15% deterioration on pulmonary artery pressure

3. Greater than 15% deterioration on airway pressure/compliance

Data from Cypel M, Yeung JC, Liu M, et al. Normothermic ex vivo lung perfusion in clinical lung transplantation. N Engl J Med 2011;364:1431–40; and Cypel M, Yeung JC, Machuca T, et al. Experience with the first 50 ex vivo lung perfusions in clinical transplantation. J Thorac Cardiovasc Surg 2012;144:1200–6.

---

possible to make a clear decision, EVLP can be extended for up to 6 hours. Lung assessment is performed in a similar manner at the fifth and sixth hours, and one extra lung radiograph is performed at 5 hours for temporal comparisons. In general, the recipient can be prepared in the operating room (OR) while the lungs are still being perfused normothermically. This strategy minimizes the second cold ischemic time.

At the time of EVLP termination, the heater/cooler is set to cool the lungs and the Fio_2 is set to 0.5. When the lungs reach 15°C, the inflow and outflow cannulas are clamped, as well as the endotracheal tube, keeping the lungs in an inflated state. The cannulas are cut from the circuit, and an antegrade flush through the PA cannula with 500 mL of Steen solution is performed. The vascular cannulas are then removed by simply cutting the Prolene sutures, and the trachea is stapled below the endotracheal tube, keeping the lung inflated. The lung is now placed in a bag filled with Perfadex, and placed on ice to be transported to the recipient OR.

Others have worked on variations of EVLP. It is important to note that there are significant differences in the techniques, equipment, and circuits from the Toronto technique. **Table 2** compares various aspects of the Toronto EVLP technique with the different methods available.

CLINICAL EXPERIENCE WITH EVLP
The Toronto Technique

The Toronto clinical experience with EVLP was reported in the *New England Journal of Medicine* in 2011 (**Table 3**).[17] The nonrandomized clinical trial included 23 donors that did not meet the conventional criteria for lung donation. In 20 cases, the physiologic performance was satisfactory and the lungs rendered 15 bilateral and 5 unilateral lung transplants. There was no difference in either the primary end point (PGD grade 2 or 3 at 72 hours) or the secondary end points (PGD 2 or 3 at intensive care unit [ICU] arrival, 24 and 48 hours; extracorporeal membrane oxygenation [ECMO] requirement; days on mechanical ventilation; ICU stay; hospital stay; and 30-day mortality) when comparing EVLP lungs with 116 contemporary non-EVLP transplants. The Toronto experience was recently updated with 58 EVLPs rendering 50 lung transplants (86% yield). Again, the outcomes were similar to 367 contemporary non-EVLP cases, with

Table 2
Comparison between different EVLP protocols

Parameter	Toronto	Lund	Organ Care System
Perfusion			
Start of perfusion	150 mL/min	100 mL/min	N/A
Target flow	40% CO	100% CO	2.5 L/min
PAP	Flow dictated	Up to 20 mm Hg	N/A
LA	Closed, 3–5 mm Hg	Open, 0 mm Hg	Open, 0 mm Hg
Perfusate	Steen solution	Steen solution + RBC hct 14%	Modified LPD solution + RBC hct 15%–25%
Perfusion time	4–6 h	Up to 2 h	Transport time
Leukocyte filter	Yes	Yes	No
Ventilation			
Mode	Volume control	Volume control	Volume control
Start	32°C	32°C	N/A
Tidal volume	7 mL/kg	5–7 mL/kg	6 mL/kg
Rate	7 bpm	20 bpm	10 bpm
PEEP	5 cm H_2O	5 cm H_2O	5 cm H_2O
Fio_2	21%	50%	N/A
Main aim	Reassess/improve	Reassess	Transport
Donor phenotype	Marginal	Marginal	Standard

Abbreviations: CO, cardiac output; hct, hematocrit; LA, left atrium; LPD, low-potassium dextran; PAP, pulmonary artery pressure; N/A, not available; RBC, red blood cell.

Modified from Sanchez PG, D'Ovidio F. Ex-vivo lung perfusion. Curr Opin Organ Transplant 2012;17:490–5.

a 2.0% incidence of PGD grade 3 at 72 hours in the study group versus 8.5% in the control cases ($P = .14$). This second publication encompassed a longer study period and, thus, allowed the observation of similar 1-year survivals: 87% for the EVLP group versus 86% for the standard group.[55]

The Toronto results were subsequently reproduced by the Vienna group. In 2012, Aigner and colleagues[56] reported 13 clinical EVLPs for donors that did not meet the standard criteria. Four cases presented poor physiologic parameters during perfusion and were, therefore, discarded (success rate 69%). All the remaining 9 cases

Table 3
Clinical experience with EVLP for donors not matching conventional criteria

Group	Technique	EVLP/Tx (N)	Transplant Rate (%)	PGD 3 at 72 h (%)	Median MV (d)	30-d Mortality (%)
Toronto[55]	Toronto	58/50	86	2	2.0	4
Vienna[56]	Toronto	13/9	69	0	2.0	0
Harefield[58]	Toronto	13/6	46	N/A	8.9	0
Milan[59]	Toronto	2/2	100	0	N/A	0
Lund[63]	Lund	9/6	66	N/A	7.9	0
Gothenburg[65]	Lund	6/6	83	0	<1.0	0

Abbreviations: d, days; MV, mechanical ventilation; N/A, not available; Tx, transplants.

underwent bilateral lung transplants, with similar early results (days on mechanical ventilation, ICU and hospital stay, and 30-day mortality) when compared with 119 standard transplants performed during the study period. Although they have followed the Toronto protocol, the time that the lungs were kept on EVLP ranged from 2 to 4 hours rather than the 4 to 6 hours reported by the latter.

The results of the combined clinical EVLP experience from Toronto, Vienna, and Paris were presented in the 2013 International Society for Heart and Lung Transplantation (ISHLT) meeting.[57] From September 2008 to August 2012, 125 clinical EVLPs were performed, with an 82.5% utilization rate. The incidence of PGD grade 3 at 72 hours was only 5%, with an 88% 1-year survival. These data reinforce the successful use of EVLP for the preservation of high-risk donor lungs.

The Harefield Hospital also reported its experience with EVLP in 13 sets of high-risk donor lungs, resulting in 6 bilateral lungs transplants (success rate 46%).[58] The perfusion times were also shorter than Toronto, with an average of 2 hours. Furthermore, in 3 of the transplanted cases, there was no interval lung radiograph examination because the group considered the initial one satisfactory. Also worth mentioning is that 2 cases of rejected lungs were caused by technical problems (one case of LA cuff that was too short and one case of inadvertent circuit misconnection). From 6 patients, 3 had an uneventful recovery, 1 developed PGD grade 2, and the remaining 2 had non–EVLP-related complications. End points, such as ICU and hospital stay and 3- and 6-month survival, were comparable with those of 86 standard transplants.

A limited experience from the Milan group was also recently reported, with 2 EVLPs resulting in 2 lung transplants with favorable outcomes.[59] Of note is that this group followed the Toronto protocol, with the exception of the supplementation of packed blood cells to the perfusion circuit.

The group from Madrid used EVLP in the setting of uncontrolled Maastricht I donors after cardiac death.[60] Following the evaluation of 8 pairs of lungs, the transplantation criteria was met in 4 cases that underwent bilateral transplantation, with no PGD grade 3.

Currently, there is an ongoing Food and Drug Administration–mandated multicenter clinical trial (Normothermic Ex Vivo Lung Perfusion as an Assessment of Extended/Marginal Donor Lungs [NOVEL] Trial) to evaluate marginal donor lungs. The preliminary data presented at the 2013 ISHLT annual meeting revealed 31 patients that received EVLP lungs with short-term outcomes (PGD, length on mechanical ventilation, ICU stay, hospital stay, and 30-day mortality) similar to 31 non-EVLP controls.[61] Definitive results should become available soon and will dictate the regulation of EVLP and its potential widespread utilization in the United States.

The Lund Technique

Using their own technique, in 2001, Steen and coworkers[62] reported the use of EVLP for short-term ex vivo perfusion to assess the lungs of a donor after cardiac death. These lungs were subsequently transplanted with good outcomes. Indeed, Steen is to be credited for initiating a revisit of the concept of EVLP in the modern era of transplantation. In 2009, the same group reported the use of EVLP for the evaluation of 9 donors with lungs initially unsuitable for transplantation.[63] This assessment resulted in 6 cases of bilateral lung transplantation. The 3-month survival was 100%; however, patients experienced a long ICU stay (median 13 days) and a median time on mechanical ventilation of 191 hours.[64] This report also proved the value of EVLP as a preservation method that can expand the donor pool in smaller programs because these 6 cases corresponded to a 35% increase over the prior transplant activity in that institution.

The group from the University of Gothenburg reported their outcomes with 6 donors initially unsuitable for lung transplantation.[65] After EVLP, 2 single lungs were declined because macroscopic evaluation revealed either edema development or persistent consolidation (one case each). The remaining lungs were allocated for 4 bilateral and 2 unilateral lung transplants. The results were favorable, with 100% 30-day survival and only one case of PGD grade 2.

The Portable Ex Vivo Technique

Although not aiming to evaluate and improve the function of donor lungs initially deemed unsuitable for transplantation, but with the primary objective of using a portable ex vivo preservation system to transport donor lungs meeting conventional criteria, the programs of Hannover and Madrid have recently reported their joint pilot study with 12 patients using the Transmedics (Andover, MA, USA) machine.[66] The average time on the perfusion/ventilation circuit was 303 minutes. All patients underwent bilateral lung transplantation; the early outcomes were favorable, with most of the patients extubated within 36 hours. At 72 hours, 4 patients presented with PGD grade 2, with the remaining being either grade 1 or 0. This pilot study proved the safety of this approach. The group is now conducting a multicenter randomized clinical trial to test if there is any benefit of further shortening cold ischemic time and having the lungs on normothermic EVLP for most of the preservation time.

THERAPEUTIC OPPORTUNITIES: EVLP AS A TARGETED INJURY-SPECIFIC TREATMENT PLATFORM
Edema

In their studies of lung physiology and the impact of alveolar fluid clearance on lung edema formation, Matthay's group has shown that human lungs rejected for transplantation and perfused ex vivo have the capability of enhancing alveolar fluid clearance from a basal of 19% per hour to 43% per hour with beta-adrenergic (airway-instilled terbutaline) stimulation.[36]

More recently, the continuous delivery of salbutamol into the perfusate for 180 minutes was shown to render better pulmonary physiology (both hemodynamics and mechanics) while on EVLP.[67] More solid conclusions could not be drawn because lungs were not transplanted. It is rather striking to note that, in this noninjury model, the control group presented a decrease of more than 50% on dynamic compliance over 4 hours of EVLP in that system.

Infection

Infection is a common concern whenever assessing a potential lung donor. Advanced infection (pneumonia) is generally a contraindication to transplantation; for the authors, it is currently a contraindication for clinical EVLP. The authors have explored the theoretical potential of EVLP to treat infected donor lungs. The EVLP circuit allows for the utilization of very-high-dose antibiotics that could not be used in vivo and also provided a very long drug half-life because the drugs are not cleared from the circuit.[68] Two important conclusions were drawn: Firstly, not all lungs deemed infected based on clinical findings by a group of experienced lung transplant surgeons actually had histologic findings of pneumonia (when subsequently evaluated by a pathologist). Secondly, most lungs treated with high-dose ex vivo antibiotics demonstrated a decreased bacterial load over time with improving lung function and without signs of pulmonary toxicity. Further work is required to determine when such lungs would be safely transplantable.

More recently, Lee and colleagues developed a model of ex vivo *Escherichia coli* pneumonia that showed significant improvements after delivery of intra-airway mesenchymal stem cells.[69] This therapy promoted the restoration of alveolar fluid clearance and potentiation of bacterial killing mechanisms. Keratinocyte growth factor secreted by mesenchymal stem cells was shown to be, at least in part, responsible for the obtained benefits.

Inflammation

Gene therapy

For more than a decade, antiinflammatory gene therapy for the donor lung has been a focus of the authors' research laboratory. The beneficial effects of adenovirus vector encoding human interleukin-10 (AdhIL-10) delivery to the donor before organ procurement have been shown experimentally.[70–73] Genetic modification of the donor lung to improve function after transplant is, thus, a proven concept.

Advanced organ therapies, such as gene therapy, were, in fact, the impetus for the development of EVLP. The concept of a system that can adequately preserve the lungs while keeping them metabolically active at normothermia possesses several advantages: (1) possibility of simple vector delivery to the donor lung at the recipient hospital site, (2) provision of an ideal time frame to potentiate transgene expression, and (3) mitigation of theoretical local and systemic host response to the vector and any vector-related toxicity. Cypel and coworkers have shown that ex vivo AdhIL-10 resulted in efficient transgene expression, which translated into better lung function and decreased levels of inflammatory cytokines both in porcine and in human lungs.[74] Moreover, they were able to show evidence of lung structural repair at the level of cytoskeleton. Yeung and colleagues[75] have reported the lack of local toxicity of ex vivo AdhIL-10 delivery, with improved lung function both during EVLP and after transplantation. The safety and efficacy of ex vivo AdhIL-10 gene therapy are currently under study in a preclinical survival model.[76]

Stem cell therapy

After demonstration of the benefits of in vivo intra-airway delivery of mesenchymal stem cells in a model of E coli endotoxin-induced lung injury, Matthay's group has explored the use of a similar approach in the ex vivo setting.[77,78] Intrabronchial delivery of mesenchymal stem cells during EVLP was shown to improve edema and inflammatory cell infiltration on histology. Moreover, mesenchymal stem cells or its culture medium restored alveolar fluid clearance to normal levels, possibly through overexpression of epithelial Na^+ channels in alveolar type II cells.

Aspiration

The potential of ex vivo treatment of lungs damaged by aspiration has been previously explored. The University of Zurich group has shown that in a model of intratracheal instillation of betaine-hydrochloride with pepsin, the administration of surfactant after initiation of EVLP rendered better pulmonary mechanics and hemodynamics when compared with lungs with no treatment.[79] Nevertheless, the short perfusion time (only 2 hours) and the lack of post-EVLP transplantation may be the reasons it failed to show clear benefits of ex vivo surfactant lavage over in vivo surfactant lavage before organ procurement.

The Leuven group developed a model of gastric acid aspiration that shows higher pulmonary vascular resistance and worsened pulmonary mechanics on the EVLP circuit as compared with sham animals.[80] In a subsequent experiment, they have studied the effects of preinjury intravenous steroids and macrolides on EVLP performance.[81] Although gas exchange was better in pigs treated with methylprednisolone, the shortened perfusion period (only 2 hours) may explain why there was no difference in terms of pulmonary mechanics, proinflammatory cytokines, and cell count on bronchoalveolar lavage and also on lung histology in animals that were treated with either steroids or macrolides compared with controls. The data available, although encouraging, are preliminary; studies on reconditioning lungs damaged by aspiration using longer perfusion periods are required to see if the benefits of surfactant treatment can be enhanced and, thus, increase the potential for clinical translation.

Pulmonary Embolism

Careful pathologic examination reveals thromboembolic disease in 35% of lungs rejected for transplantation.[82] More importantly, in those lungs actually used, either blood clots or fat emboli were observed in 31% during the retrograde flush.[83] This finding was associated with higher rates of severe PGD. To further address the theoretical thrombotic complications of lung donation after cardiac death, Inci and colleagues[84] added urokinase to perfusate during 90 minutes of EVLP. Although parameters did not improve to the level of conventional heart-beating donors, pulmonary vascular resistance, gas exchange, wet-to-dry ratio, and histology were better than the cardiac death group perfused without thrombolytics.

The use of EVLP as a preservation technique to deliver thrombolytics and treat pulmonary clot, whether embolic or thrombotic in nature, seems logical: (1) It provides time while keeping the lungs active and stable. (2) The continuous hemodynamic monitoring provides a tool to evaluate the therapeutic response in cases of massive/submassive embolism. (3) The absence of liver and plasma in the circuit greatly downregulates clearance mechanisms. (4) The accumulation of fibrinolytics in the interstitial space with theoretical toxicity after reperfusion is proven to be minimal. (5) The last antegrade flush after EVLP termination clears the medication from the circulation.[85–87] The authors' group recently illustrated this concept after the successful transplantation of lungs with massive pulmonary embolism treated with thrombolytics delivered during EVLP.[88]

Donation After Cardiac Death

The retrieval of lungs from DCD donors represents a significant potential source of donor organs. By the very nature of the events, Maastricht category 1 and 2 donor lungs represent a higher risk with inadequate opportunities to fully assess the organ and, hence, are ideally suited to be assessed and treated by EVLP.

Category 3 and 4 donor lungs are potentially superior organs to organs retrieved from donors after brain death because they have not been subjected to the deleterious effects of brain death in the donor. However, some of these lungs are still at risk because these donors represent a spectrum and many are near brain death or would meet the criteria if reassessed neurologically. More importantly, the process of withdrawing life support adds additional potential risk of injury to the donor lung, that is, of shock lung from prolonged agonal hypotension or aspiration after removal of the endotracheal tube.[89] Therefore, a donor lung that started out good may not end up being suitable after the process of withdrawal of life support in the DCD donor. This area is of considerable debate in the field.

Initially applied to reassess lungs from donors after cardiac death, EVLP has been extensively studied as a platform to improve this particular subset of lungs.[62] In the setting of uncontrolled cardiac death, Nakajima and coworkers[90] evaluated the beneficial effects of nitroglycerin and dibutyryl cyclic adenosine monophosphate added to Steen solution during 3.5 hours of EVLP for lungs submitted to 4 hours of warm ischemia.[90] EVLP lungs had better function posttransplantation, with a lower histologic grade of acute lung injury and lesser formation of microthrombi when compared with lungs without EVLP.

Sanchez and coworkers[91] have studied the importance of adding heparin to a DCD protocol. Pigs with and without heparin preinduction of cardiac arrest were submitted to 1 hour of warm ischemia followed by 6 hours of cold ischemia before being assessed by EVLP. In the heparin group, EVLP physiology (gas exchange, compliance, pulmonary vascular resistance, bronchoalveolar lavage protein content, wet-to-dry ratio, and Na^+-K^+ ATPase activity) was significantly better than in the non-heparin group. Furthermore, aggregated platelets and fibrin deposition were evident in the latter group after 1 hour of warm ischemia.

Egan's laboratory[92,93] has focused research efforts on DCDs for a long time. In 2 separate EVLP studies, they evaluated the effects of airway delivery of nitric oxide and, more recently, of carbon monoxide during 1 hour of warm ischemia, 15 minutes of EVLP, and finally in the recipient after reperfusion. Both of these agents were beneficial and provided better lung function and less edema formation after transplantation.[92,93]

Mulloy and coworkers[94] have recently reported interesting results. In a model of 1 hour of warm ischemia in pigs, lung function after 4 hours of EVLP and after 4 hours of transplantation was significantly better when EVLP was preceded by 4 hours of cold static preservation as opposed to immediate EVLP. Furthermore, lungs in the delayed EVLP group presented lower levels of proinflammatory cytokines on bronchoalveolar lavage and also lower histologic lung injury scores. The investigators hypothesized that a period of hypothermia may have been advantageous in the sense that it arrested ongoing deleterious mechanisms of warm ischemic injury before the initiation of EVLP. Further studies are required to better understand this intriguing finding.

The growing amount of research dedicated to donation after cardiac death summarized here clearly highlights the potential of EVLP as a platform not only to assess but also to deliver therapies to improve lungs from this particular subset of donors.

THE FUTURE
Specialized EVLP Centers

Because EVLP requires not only technological resources but also significant personnel expertise, the establishment of specialized centers to serve regional demands seems reasonable. These centers would ideally take advantage of their geographically favorable locations and be able to perform EVLP for organ assessment and reconditioning in a large scale. Once transplantation criteria are achieved, these organs would be sent to the satellite centers.

This concept is better illustrated by a recent report by Wigfield and coworkers.[95] A donor became available for an emergently listed patient at the Loyola University Medical Center. However, after the initial assessment, it was clear that the donor was too high risk for lung transplantation. The team at the University of Toronto was, thus, contacted and, after receiving the lungs and performing EVLP for 4 hours, was able to reassure physiologic improvement and transplantability. The lungs were sent back to Illinois and successfully transplanted into a 54-year-old recipient on venovenous ECMO.

Biomarkers in EVLP

Prolonged EVLP has opened an important door for diagnosis and treatment of the donor lung in a personalized fashion. Although the current practice of EVLP relies largely on physiologic assessment with conventional monitoring, the authors think that more sophisticated tools will allow accurate ex vivo bio-profiling of the donor lung. Although several biomarkers have been linked to PGD, EVLP has brought a unique situation: For the first time, this valuable information will be available hours before lung implantation and will be part of the decision-making process.[96,97] Rapid diagnostic modalities coupled with transplantomics will be instrumental to bring this concept to reality.[98–100] Furthermore, because lungs can be safely preserved for prolonged periods, these biomarkers can also potentially be repeatedly used for lung reassessment after the delivery of targeted therapies, ultimately dictating lung transplantability.

SUMMARY

EVLP has been further refined and developed as a functional organ preservation technique that maintains the lungs stable for prolonged periods under normothermia. After extensive experimental research, it has been successfully translated into clinical practice, with a growing number of centers worldwide reporting favorable outcomes. More than keeping the lungs stable, EVLP provides the opportunity to deliver personalized medicine for the organ, that is, the opportunity to define the specific diagnosis and deliver appropriate specific treatment to a metabolically active organ. The authors envision the future of EVLP with the establishment of specialized EVLP centers that are able to provide large-scale advanced organ treatment and repair, using advanced rapid diagnostic tools to guide the delivery of personalized medicine to the donor organ.

REFERENCES

1. Christie JD, Edwards LB, Kucheryavaya AY, et al. The Registry of the International Society for Heart and Lung Transplantation: 29th adult lung and heart-lung transplant report-2012. J Heart Lung Transplant 2012;31:1073–86.
2. Valapour M, Paulson K, Smith JM, et al. OPTN/SRTR 2011 annual data report: lung. Am J Transplant 2013;13(Suppl 1):149–77.
3. Titman A, Rogers CA, Bonser RS, et al. Disease-specific survival benefit of lung transplantation in adults: a national cohort study. Am J Transplant 2009;9:1640–9.
4. Klein AS, Messersmith EE, Ratner LE, et al. Organ donation and utilization in the United States, 1999–2008. Am J Transplant 2010;10:973–86.
5. Botha P, Trivedi D, Weir CJ, et al. Extended donor criteria in lung transplantation: impact on organ allocation. J Thorac Cardiovasc Surg 2006;131:1154–60.
6. Pierre AF, Sekine Y, Hutcheon M, et al. Evaluation of extended donor and recipient criteria for lung transplantation. J Heart Lung Transplant 2001;20:256.
7. D'Alessandro AM, Hoffmann RM, Knechtle SJ, et al. Successful extrarenal transplantation from non-heart-beating donors. Transplantation 1995;59:977–82.
8. Cypel M, Sato M, Yildirim E, et al. Initial experience with lung donation after cardiocirculatory death in Canada. J Heart Lung Transplant 2009;28:753–8.
9. Erasmus ME, Verschuuren EA, Nijkamp DM, et al. Lung transplantation from nonheparinized category III non-heart-beating donors. A single-centre report. Transplantation 2010;89:452–7.
10. Love RB. Perspectives on lung transplantation and donation-after-determination-of-cardiac-death donors. Am J Transplant 2012;12:2271–2.
11. Mason DP, Brown CR, Murthy SC, et al. Growing single-center experience with lung transplantation using donation after cardiac death. Ann Thorac Surg 2012;94:406–11 [discussion: 11–2].

12. De Oliveira NC, Osaki S, Maloney JD, et al. Lung transplantation with donation after cardiac death donors: long-term follow-up in a single center. J Thorac Cardiovasc Surg 2010;139:1306–15.

13. Levvey BJ, Harkess M, Hopkins P, et al. Excellent clinical outcomes from a national donation-after-determination-of-cardiac-death lung transplant collaborative. Am J Transplant 2012;12:2406–13.

14. Puri V, Scavuzzo M, Guthrie T, et al. Lung transplantation and donation after cardiac death: a single center experience. Ann Thorac Surg 2009;88:1609–14 [discussion: 14–5].

15. de Antonio DG, Marcos R, Laporta R, et al. Results of clinical lung transplant from uncontrolled non-heart-beating donors. J Heart Lung Transplant 2007;26:529–34.

16. Bonser RS, Taylor R, Collett D, et al. Effect of donor smoking on survival after lung transplantation: a cohort study of a prospective registry. Lancet 2012;380:747–55.

17. Cypel M, Yeung JC, Liu M, et al. Normothermic ex vivo lung perfusion in clinical lung transplantation. N Engl J Med 2011;364:1431–40.

18. Boutilier RG. Mechanisms of cell survival in hypoxia and hypothermia. J Exp Biol 2001;204:3171–81.

19. Zhao G, al-Mehdi AB, Fisher AB. Anoxia-reoxygenation versus ischemia in isolated rat lungs. Am J Physiol 1997;273:L1112–7.

20. Hochachka PW. Defense strategies against hypoxia and hypothermia. Science 1986;231:234–41.

21. Keshavjee SH, Yamazaki F, Cardoso PF, et al. A method for safe twelve-hour pulmonary preservation. J Thorac Cardiovasc Surg 1989;98:529–34.

22. Maccherini M, Keshavjee SH, Slutsky AS, et al. The effect of low-potassium-dextran versus Euro-Collins solution for preservation of isolated type II pneumocytes. Transplantation 1991;52:621–6.

23. Keshavjee SH, Yamazaki F, Yokomise H, et al. The role of dextran 40 and potassium in extended hypothermic lung preservation for transplantation. J Thorac Cardiovasc Surg 1992;103:314–25.

24. Haverich A, Aziz S, Scott WC, et al. Improved lung preservation using Euro-Collins solution for flush-perfusion. Thorac Cardiovasc Surg 1986;34:368–76.

25. Wang LS, Nakamoto K, Hsieh CM, et al. Influence of temperature of flushing solution on lung preservation. Ann Thorac Surg 1993;55:711–5.

26. Albes JM, Fischer F, Bando T, et al. Influence of the perfusate temperature on lung preservation: is there an optimum? Eur Surg Res 1997;29:5–11.

27. Date H, Lima O, Matsumura A, et al. In a canine model, lung preservation at 10 degrees C is superior to that at 4 degrees C. A comparison of two preservation temperatures on lung function and on adenosine triphosphate level measured by phosphorus 31-nuclear magnetic resonance. J Thorac Cardiovasc Surg 1992;103:773–80.

28. Date H, Matsumura A, Manchester JK, et al. Changes in alveolar oxygen and carbon dioxide concentration and oxygen consumption during lung preservation. The maintenance of aerobic metabolism during lung preservation. J Thorac Cardiovasc Surg 1993;105:492–501.

29. Fukuse T, Hirata T, Nakamura T, et al. Influence of deflated and anaerobic conditions during cold storage on rat lungs. Am J Respir Crit Care Med 1999;160:621–7.

30. Struber M, Hohlfeld JM, Kofidis T, et al. Surfactant function in lung transplantation after 24 hours of ischemia: advantage of retrograde flush perfusion for preservation. J Thorac Cardiovasc Surg 2002;123:98–103.

31. de Perrot M, Keshavjee S. Lung preservation. Semin Thorac Cardiovasc Surg 2004;16:300–8.

32. de Perrot M, Keshavjee S. Lung transplantation. Lung preservation. Chest Surg Clin N Am 2003;13:443–62.
33. Carrel A, Lindbergh CA. The culture of whole organs. Science 1935;81:621–3.
34. Cypel M, Rubacha M, Yeung J, et al. Normothermic ex vivo perfusion prevents lung injury compared to extended cold preservation for transplantation. Am J Transplant 2009;9:2262–9.
35. Cypel M, Yeung JC, Hirayama S, et al. Technique for prolonged normothermic ex vivo lung perfusion. J Heart Lung Transplant 2008;27:1319–25.
36. Frank JA, Briot R, Lee JW, et al. Physiological and biochemical markers of alveolar epithelial barrier dysfunction in perfused human lungs. Am J Physiol Lung Cell Mol Physiol 2007;293:L52–9.
37. Sakuma T, Okaniwa G, Nakada T, et al. Alveolar fluid clearance in the resected human lung. Am J Respir Crit Care Med 1994;150:305–10.
38. Broccard AF, Hotchkiss JR, Kuwayama N, et al. Consequences of vascular flow on lung injury induced by mechanical ventilation. Am J Respir Crit Care Med 1998;157:1935–42.
39. Piacentini E, Lopez-Aguilar J, Garcia-Martin C, et al. Effects of vascular flow and PEEP in a multiple hit model of lung injury in isolated perfused rabbit lungs. J Trauma 2008;65:147–53.
40. Fisher AB, Dodia C, Linask J. Perfusate composition and edema formation in isolated rat lungs. Exp Lung Res 1980;1:13–21.
41. Rubini A. Effect of perfusate temperature on pulmonary vascular resistance and compliance by arterial and venous occlusion in the rat. Eur J Appl Physiol 2005; 93:435–9.
42. Suzuki S, Sugita M, Ono S, et al. Difference in the effects of low temperatures on the tension of human pulmonary artery and vein ring segments. Respiration 2000;67:189–93.
43. Pierre AF, DeCampos KN, Liu M, et al. Rapid reperfusion causes stress failure in ischemic rat lungs. J Thorac Cardiovasc Surg 1998;116:932–42.
44. Broccard AF, Vannay C, Feihl F, et al. Impact of low pulmonary vascular pressure on ventilator-induced lung injury. Crit Care Med 2002;30:2183–90.
45. Petak F, Habre W, Hantos Z, et al. Effects of pulmonary vascular pressures and flow on airway and parenchymal mechanics in isolated rat lungs. J Appl Physiol 2002;92:169–78.
46. Chang RS, Wright K, Effros RM. Role of albumin in prevention of edema in perfused rabbit lungs. J Appl Physiol 1981;50:1065–70.
47. Kraft SA, Fujishima S, McGuire GP, et al. Effect of blood and albumin on pulmonary hypertension and edema in perfused rabbit lungs. J Appl Physiol 1995;78: 499–504.
48. Laumonier T, Walpen AJ, Maurus CF, et al. Dextran sulfate acts as an endothelial cell protectant and inhibits human complement and natural killer cell-mediated cytotoxicity against porcine cells. Transplantation 2003;76:838–43.
49. Zeerleder S, Mauron T, Lammle B, et al. Effect of low-molecular weight dextran sulfate on coagulation and platelet function tests. Thromb Res 2002;105: 441–6.
50. Fischer S, Matte-Martyn A, De Perrot M, et al. Low-potassium dextran preservation solution improves lung function after human lung transplantation. J Thorac Cardiovasc Surg 2001;121:594–6.
51. Ventilation with lower tidal volumes as compared with traditional tidal volumes for acute lung injury and the acute respiratory distress syndrome. The Acute Respiratory Distress Syndrome Network. N Engl J Med 2000;342:1301–8.

52. Amato MB, Barbas CS, Medeiros DM, et al. Effect of a protective-ventilation strategy on mortality in the acute respiratory distress syndrome. N Engl J Med 1998;338:347–54.
53. de Perrot M, Imai Y, Volgyesi GA, et al. Effect of ventilator-induced lung injury on the development of reperfusion injury in a rat lung transplant model. J Thorac Cardiovasc Surg 2002;124:1137–44.
54. Yeung JC, Cypel M, Machuca TN, et al. Physiologic assessment of the ex vivo donor lung for transplantation. J Heart Lung Transplant 2012;31:1120–6.
55. Cypel M, Yeung JC, Machuca T, et al. Experience with the first 50 ex vivo lung perfusions in clinical transplantation. J Thorac Cardiovasc Surg 2012;144:1200–6.
56. Aigner C, Slama A, Hotzenecker K, et al. Clinical ex vivo lung perfusion–pushing the limits. Am J Transplant 2012;12:1839–47.
57. Cypel M, Aigner C, Sage E, et al. Three center experience with clinical normothermic ex vivo lung perfusion. J Heart Lung Transplant 2013;32:S16.
58. Zych B, Popov AF, Stavri G, et al. Early outcomes of bilateral sequential single lung transplantation after ex-vivo lung evaluation and reconditioning. J Heart Lung Transplant 2012;31:274–81.
59. Valenza F, Rosso L, Gatti S, et al. Extracorporeal lung perfusion and ventilation to improve donor lung function and increase the number of organs available for transplantation. Transplant Proc 2012;44:1826–9.
60. Moradiellos FJ, Naranjo JM, Cordoba M, et al. Clinical lung transplantation after ex vivo evaluation of uncontrolled non heart-beating donor lungs: initial experience. J Heart Lung Transplant 2011;30:S38.
61. Sanchez PG, Davis RD, D'Ovidio F, et al. Normothermic ex vivo lung perfusion as an assessment of marginal donor lungs-the NOVEL lung trial. J Heart Lung Transplant 2013;32:S16–7.
62. Steen S, Sjoberg T, Pierre L, et al. Transplantation of lungs from a non-heart-beating donor. Lancet 2001;357:825–9.
63. Ingemansson R, Eyjolfsson A, Mared L, et al. Clinical transplantation of initially rejected donor lungs after reconditioning ex vivo. Ann Thorac Surg 2009;87:255–60.
64. Lindstedt S, Eyjolfsson A, Koul B, et al. How to recondition ex vivo initially rejected donor lungs for clinical transplantation: clinical experience from Lund University Hospital. Am J Transplant 2011;2011:754383.
65. Wallinder A, Ricksten SE, Hansson C, et al. Transplantation of initially rejected donor lungs after ex vivo lung perfusion. J Thorac Cardiovasc Surg 2012;144:1222–8.
66. Warnecke G, Moradiellos J, Tudorache I, et al. Normothermic perfusion of donor lungs for preservation and assessment with the Organ Care System Lung before bilateral transplantation: a pilot study of 12 patients. Lancet 2012;380:1851–8.
67. Valenza F, Rosso L, Coppola S, et al. Beta-adrenergic agonist infusion during extracorporeal lung perfusion: effects on glucose concentration in the perfusion fluid and on lung function. J Heart Lung Transplant 2012;31:524–30.
68. Bonato R, Machuca T, Cypel M, et al. Ex vivo treatment of infection in human donor lungs. J Heart Lung Transplant 2012;31:S97–8.
69. Lee JW, Krasnodembskaya A, McKenna DH, et al. Therapeutic effects of human mesenchymal stem cells in ex vivo human lungs injured with live bacteria. Am J Respir Crit Care Med 2013;187(7):751–60.
70. Fischer S, Liu M, MacLean AA, et al. In vivo transtracheal adenovirus-mediated transfer of human interleukin-10 gene to donor lungs ameliorates

ischemia-reperfusion injury and improves early posttransplant graft function in the rat. Hum Gene Ther 2001;12:1513–26.

71. Martins S, de Perrot M, Imai Y, et al. Transbronchial administration of adenoviral-mediated interleukin-10 gene to the donor improves function in a pig lung transplant model. Gene Ther 2004;11:1786–96.

72. Fischer S, De Perrot M, Liu M, et al. Interleukin 10 gene transfection of donor lungs ameliorates posttransplant cell death by a switch from cellular necrosis to apoptosis. J Thorac Cardiovasc Surg 2003;126:1174–80.

73. Cassivi SD, Cardella JA, Fischer S, et al. Transtracheal gene transfection of donor lungs prior to organ procurement increases transgene levels at reperfusion and following transplantation. J Heart Lung Transplant 1999;18:1181–8.

74. Cypel M, Liu M, Rubacha M, et al. Functional repair of human donor lungs by IL-10 gene therapy. Sci Transl Med 2009;1:4ra9.

75. Yeung JC, Wagnetz D, Cypel M, et al. Ex vivo adenoviral vector gene delivery results in decreased vector-associated inflammation pre- and post-lung transplantation in the pig. Mol Ther 2012;20:1204–11.

76. Machuca T, Bonato R, Cypel M, et al. Ex vivo adenoviral IL-10 gene therapy in a pig lung transplantation survival model. J Heart Lung Transplant 2012;31:S141.

77. Lee JW, Fang X, Gupta N, et al. Allogeneic human mesenchymal stem cells for treatment of E. coli endotoxin-induced acute lung injury in the ex vivo perfused human lung. Proc Natl Acad Sci U S A 2009;106:16357–62.

78. Gupta N, Su X, Popov B, et al. Intrapulmonary delivery of bone marrow-derived mesenchymal stem cells improves survival and attenuates endotoxin-induced acute lung injury in mice. J Immunol 2007;179:1855–63.

79. Inci I, Ampollini L, Arni S, et al. Ex vivo reconditioning of marginal donor lungs injured by acid aspiration. J Heart Lung Transplant 2008;27:1229–36.

80. Meers CM, Tsagkaropoulos S, Wauters S, et al. A model of ex vivo perfusion of porcine donor lungs injured by gastric aspiration: a step towards pretransplant reconditioning. J Surg Res 2011;170:e159–67.

81. Meers CM, Wauters S, Verbeken E, et al. Preemptive therapy with steroids but not macrolides improves gas exchange in caustic-injured donor lungs. J Surg Res 2011;170:e141–8.

82. Ware LB, Fang X, Wang Y, et al. High prevalence of pulmonary arterial thrombi in donor lungs rejected for transplantation. J Heart Lung Transplant 2005;24:1650–6.

83. Oto T, Rabinov M, Griffiths AP, et al. Unexpected donor pulmonary embolism affects early outcomes after lung transplantation: a major mechanism of primary graft failure? J Thorac Cardiovasc Surg 2005;130:1446.

84. Inci I, Zhai W, Arni S, et al. Fibrinolytic treatment improves the quality of lungs retrieved from non-heart-beating donors. J Heart Lung Transplant 2007;26:1054–60.

85. Chandler WL, Alessi MC, Aillaud MF, et al. Clearance of tissue plasminogen activator (TPA) and TPA/plasminogen activator inhibitor type 1 (PAI-1) complex: relationship to elevated TPA antigen in patients with high PAI-1 activity levels. Circulation 1997;96:761–8.

86. Dalla-Volta S, Palla A, Santolicandro A, et al. PAIMS 2: alteplase combined with heparin versus heparin in the treatment of acute pulmonary embolism. Plasminogen activator Italian multicenter study 2. J Am Coll Cardiol 1992;20:520–6.

87. Meneveau N, Schiele F, Metz D, et al. Comparative efficacy of a two-hour regimen of streptokinase versus alteplase in acute massive pulmonary

embolism: immediate clinical and hemodynamic outcome and one-year follow-up. J Am Coll Cardiol 1998;31:1057–63.

88. Machuca TN, Hsin MK, Ott HC, et al. Injury specific treatment of the donor lung: pulmonary thrombolysis followed by successful lung transplantation. Am J Respir Crit Care Med, in press.

89. Tremblay LN, Yamashiro T, DeCampos KN, et al. Effect of hypotension preceding death on the function of lungs from donors with nonbeating hearts. J Heart Lung Transplant 1996;15:260–8.

90. Nakajima D, Chen F, Yamada T, et al. Reconditioning of lungs donated after circulatory death with normothermic ex vivo lung perfusion. J Heart Lung Transplant 2012;31:187–93.

91. Sanchez PG, Bittle GJ, Williams K, et al. Ex vivo lung evaluation of prearrest heparinization in donation after cardiac death. Ann Surg 2013;257:534–41.

92. Dong B, Stewart PW, Egan TM. Postmortem and ex vivo carbon monoxide ventilation reduces injury in rat lungs transplanted from non-heart-beating donors. J Thorac Cardiovasc Surg 2013;146(2):429–36.e1.

93. Dong BM, Abano JB, Egan TM. Nitric oxide ventilation of rat lungs from non-heart-beating donors improves posttransplant function. Am J Transplant 2009; 9:2707–15.

94. Mulloy DP, Stone ML, Crosby IK, et al. Ex vivo rehabilitation of non-heart-beating donor lungs in preclinical porcine model: delayed perfusion results in superior lung function. J Thorac Cardiovasc Surg 2012;144:1208–15.

95. Wigfield CH, Cypel M, Yeung J, et al. Successful emergent lung transplantation after remote ex vivo perfusion optimization and transportation of donor lungs. Am J Transplant 2012;12:2838–44.

96. De Perrot M, Sekine Y, Fischer S, et al. Interleukin-8 release during early reperfusion predicts graft function in human lung transplantation. Am J Respir Crit Care Med 2002;165:211–5.

97. Hoffman SA, Wang L, Shah CV, et al. Plasma cytokines and chemokines in primary graft dysfunction post-lung transplantation. Am J Transplant 2009;9: 389–96.

98. Sarwal MM, Benjamin J, Butte AJ, et al. Transplantomics and biomarkers in organ transplantation: a report from the first international conference. Transplantation 2011;91:379–82.

99. Soleymani L, Fang Z, Sargent EH, et al. Programming the detection limits of biosensors through controlled nanostructuring. Nat Nanotechnol 2009;4:844–8.

100. Yang H, Hui A, Pampalakis G, et al. Direct, electronic microRNA detection for the rapid determination of differential expression profiles. Angew Chem Int Ed Engl 2009;48:8461–4.

The Kidney Allocation System

John J. Friedewald, MD[a],*, Ciara J. Samana, MSPH[b],
Bertram L. Kasiske, MD[c,d], Ajay K. Israni, MD, MS[c,d,e],
Darren Stewart, MS[b], Wida Cherikh, PhD[b],
Richard N. Formica, MD[f,g]

KEYWORDS

• Kidney transplant • Organ allocation • Transplant waiting list

KEY POINTS

• The current kidney allocation system is outdated and has not evolved to reflect the changing demographics of patients on the waiting list.
• Without additional donor kidneys, any change in the allocation system shifts kidneys between different patient groups.
• Any changes in the allocation system will be trade-offs between equity and utility.
• The new proposed system will significantly reduce mismatches between possible donor kidney longevity and life expectancy of recipients.

Continued

This work was conducted under the auspices of the Minneapolis Medical Research Foundation, contractor for the Scientific Registry of Transplant Recipients, as a deliverable under contract no. HHSH250201000018C (US Department of Health and Human Services, Health Resources and Services Administration, Healthcare Systems Bureau, Division of Transplantation). As a US Government-sponsored work, there are no restrictions on its use. The views expressed herein are those of the authors and not necessarily those of the US Government. This work was supported wholly or in part by Health Resources and Services Administration contract 234-2005-370011C. The content is the responsibility of the authors alone and does not necessarily reflect the views or policies of the Department of Health and Human Services, nor does mention of trade names, commercial products, or organizations imply endorsement by the US Government.
The authors have nothing to disclose.
The new kidney allocation policy was approved by the Organ Procurement and Transplantation Network Board of Directors on July 25, 2013. See http://optn.transplant.hrsa.gov/PoliciesandBylaws2/policies/pdfs/policy_7.pdf.

[a] Comprehensive Transplant Center, Department of Surgery, Feinberg School of Medicine, Northwestern University, 676 North Saint Clair Street, Suite 1900, Chicago, IL 60611, USA; [b] United Network for Organ Sharing, 700 North 4th Street, Richmond, VA 23238, USA; [c] Scientific Registry of Transplant Recipients, Minneapolis Medical Research Foundation, 701 Park Avenue, Minneapolis, MN 55415-1829, USA; [d] Division of Nephrology, Department of Medicine, Hennepin County Medical Center, 701 Park Avenue, Minneapolis, MN 55415-1829, USA; [e] Department of Epidemiology and Community Health, School of Public Health, University of Minnesota, Mayo Building, A302, Mail Code 197, 420 Delaware Street Southeast, Minneapolis, MN 55455, USA; [f] Department of Internal Medicine, Yale School of Medicine, PO Box 208029, 333 Cedar Street, New Haven, CT 06520-8029, USA; [g] Department of Surgery, Yale University School of Medicine, 333 Cedar Street, New Haven, CT 06520-8029, USA
* Corresponding author.
E-mail address: jfriedew@nmh.org

Continued
- The new system more appropriately incorporates the biology of highly sensitized patients into the waiting-time scoring algorithm.
- The new system makes incremental advances toward more geographic sharing.

INTRODUCTION

Dialysis and kidney transplant are the two available active treatment options for the nearly 500,000 individuals in the United States with end-stage renal disease (ESRD). Many patients with ESRD will achieve improved quality and increased quantity of life from a kidney transplant in comparison with maintenance dialysis (**Fig. 1**).[1–3] ESRD patients can receive a kidney for transplant from a living or a recently deceased donor. The current system for allocation of deceased donor kidneys in the United States has been in place for nearly 3 decades. During this time the demand for kidney transplants has increased dramatically while the supply has remained fairly constant (**Fig. 2**). Moreover, as the criteria for eligibility for kidney transplants have broadened, the system for allocating kidneys has remained largely unchanged. This situation has resulted in ever increasing waiting times for patients as well as a patchwork of allocation variances designed to address perceived or actual deficiencies. The resulting system of allocation fails to address the differences in wait-listed patients or optimize the use of recovered organs, and is both cumbersome to administer and nearly impossible to modify. As established in the National Organ Transplant Act, the Organ Procurement and Transplantation Network (OPTN) administers the waiting list and develops policy regarding the allocation of deceased donor kidneys.[4] The OPTN contract is currently held by United Network for Organ Sharing.

LIMITATIONS OF THE CURRENT KIDNEY ALLOCATION SYSTEM

Because of the extreme mismatch between the number of listed candidates and the number of organs available for transplant (see **Fig. 2**), candidates must wait ever longer

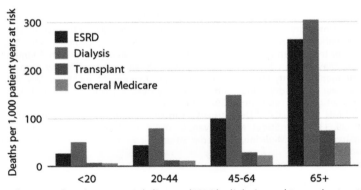

Fig. 1. Death rates of end-stage renal disease (ESRD), dialysis, and transplant patients, and in the general Medicare population, by age.

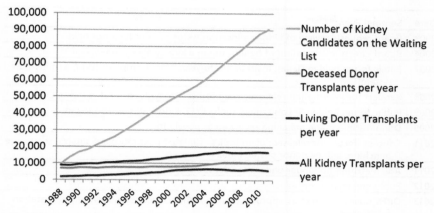

Fig. 2. Kidney transplant waiting list and numbers of transplants performed.

to receive an organ offer. Over time, as the disparity between supply of and demand for organs for transplant has grown, waiting time has become the dominant factor in allocation, surpassing the contribution of biological allocation system criteria, such as degree of immune system sensitization or degree of human leukocyte antigen (HLA) matching. As a result, this allocation system achieves only one goal: performing transplants in candidates who have waited the longest. It does not strive to improve outcomes after transplant, or to reduce mortality on the waiting list. It also fails to account for the fact that survival while on the waiting list is not the same for all candidates.

The main limitations of the current system are:

- Higher than necessary discard rates of kidneys that could benefit candidates on the waiting list
- Variability in access to transplant by candidate blood type and geographic location
- Many kidneys with more potential longevity being allocated to candidates with significantly less potential longevity and vice versa, resulting in unrealized graft years and unnecessarily high retransplant rates
- Inability to make timely modifications to the allocation system in an economical way

A CALL FOR CHANGE

In 2003, the OPTN Board of Directors charged the Kidney Transplantation Committee with reviewing the current kidney allocation policy to identify system limitations and approaches for improvement. For almost 10 years, the Committee worked to develop improved methods for kidney allocation. Two public forums have taken place, in 2007 in Dallas and in 2009 in St Louis (see sentinel events listed below). During these forums, the committee received feedback from interested parties and incorporated recommendations into iterations of its proposal. In addition, the committee circulated a concept paper that detailed various components of a kidney allocation system for discussion and consideration by the transplant community and the general public. This process culminated in the most recent version of the kidney allocation proposal, which was circulated for formal public comment in September 2012.

Date	Sentinel Event
2003	Board requests review of kidney allocation system; public hearings held
2004	Board directs investigation of benefit use in a kidney allocation system
2007	Public forum held in Dallas; main topic life-years from transplant (LYFT, a utility-based system)
2008	Request for information released; main topics kidney donor profile index, LYFT
2009	Public forum held in St Louis; main topics LYFT, kidney donor profile index
2009	Donor/recipient age matching reviewed as possibility
2011	Concept document released; main topics estimated posttransplant survival score, age matching, kidney donor profile index
2011	Age matching no longer under consideration
2012	Public comment proposal
2013	OPTN Board of Directors approves revised kidney allocation policy; implementation forthcoming

SYSTEM GOALS

By design, each organ allocation system attempts to achieve different goals. For example, the liver allocation system was modified in 2002 to allocate livers based on a candidate's probability of dying while on the waiting list. Candidates whose probability of death is higher are offered livers ahead of candidates whose probability is lower. Lungs are allocated similarly, but the lung allocation system takes into account a candidate's chance of dying while on the waiting list and during the first year following transplant.

The design of any allocation system that distributes a scare resource, such as deceased donor organs, must be based on sound ethical principles. The 2 principles primarily at work in the design of an allocation system are utility and equity (justice).[5] An allocation system that focuses on improving outcomes is considered a utility-based system, and a system that prioritizes equal access regardless of need is an equity-based system. These 2 approaches represent the polar ends of the ethical methods used to allocate a scarce resource. In organ allocation, an approach that uses the principle of utility attempts to maximize a desired outcome, such as patient or graft survival, whereas an approach that uses the principle of equity is designed to achieve fairness, which may occur at the expense of outcomes or utility measures. Ideally, everyone who needs a kidney transplant would receive a high-quality kidney and would not have to wait for it. However, the shortage of kidney donors and the changing demographics of candidates on the waiting list have become so extreme in some areas of the country (**Fig. 3**) that achieving equipoise between the principles of equity and utility is becoming ever more difficult. If kidney allocation were more heavily weighted toward achieving equity, utility measures such as life-years after transplant would decline. Alternatively, if kidney allocation were more heavily weighted toward achieving utility (defined here as life-years after transplant), equity measures such as number of transplants received by older candidates would decline (**Fig. 4**). Any redesign of the kidney allocation system must take into account the tension between equity and utility; it must balance access to transplant for everyone who could benefit across the age spectrum while maximizing the benefits of a scarce resource, the donated kidney.

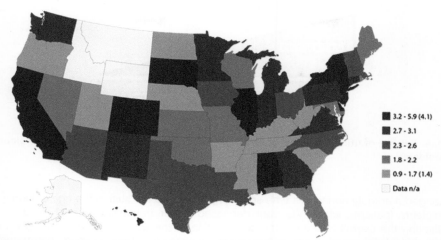

Fig. 3. Patients aged 18 years or older undergoing first-time deceased donor kidney-only transplant in 2010. Unadjusted median waiting times (years) by state of transplant center. (*From* United States Renal Data System. USRDS 2012 annual data report: atlas of chronic kidney disease and end-stage renal disease in the United States. Bethesda (MD): National Institutes of Health, National Institute of Diabetes and Digestive and Kidney Diseases; 2012.)

The following guiding principles were used to redesign the kidney allocation system. These principles were developed in consultation with transplant professionals, patients, donor family members, and members of the general public:

Proposed Goals of New Allocation System	Ethical Principle Addressed
More accurately estimate graft and recipient longevity to maximize the potential survival of every transplanted kidney and to provide acceptable levels of access for candidates on the waiting list	Utility/Equity
Promote posttransplant kidney function for candidates with the longest estimated posttransplant survival who are also the most likely to require additional transplants because of early age of ESRD onset	Utility
Minimize loss of potential functioning years of deceased donor kidney grafts through improved matching	Utility
Improve offer system efficiency and organ use through the introduction of a new scale for kidney quality, the kidney donor profile index	Utility
Reduce differences in transplant access for populations described in the National Organ Transplant Act (eg, candidates from racial/ethnic minority groups, pediatric candidates, and sensitized candidates)	Equity

COMPOSITION OF THE WAITING LIST

The candidate waiting list has grown steadily over the last several decades (see **Fig. 2**), reaching 95,459 candidates in March 2013. Beyond the sheer number of candidates, the demographics of the waiting list, particularly with respect to age, have

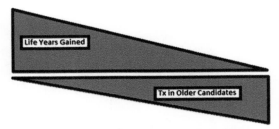

Fig. 4. Balance of utility (life-years gained) and equity (transplants [Tx] performed in older candidates).

changed markedly during this time span. **Fig. 5** depicts the shift in the age of kidney recipients (patients who underwent deceased donor transplant) over 2 decades, reflecting the overall change in the composition of the waiting list. For example, in 1990, 3% of deceased donor kidney recipients were older than 65 years, compared with 16% in 2009. Similar increases occurred regarding transplants in recipients older than 50 years, whereas transplants in recipients aged 18 to 50 years steadily decreased. Pediatric candidates receive separate priority on the list and therefore have not been affected by changes in wait-list composition. The aging of candidates on the waiting list poses challenges not only in allocation of organs but also in caring for recipients before and after transplant. The overall distribution of candidates and donors, based on age, is shown in **Fig. 6**.

ESTIMATED POSTTRANSPLANT SURVIVAL

A tool to estimate the anticipated posttransplant survival of a patient receiving a kidney transplant was developed to help improve the allocation system.[6] By design, this tool uses only 4 variables to stratify patients based on predicted survival: recipient age, diabetic status, time on dialysis, and number of prior solid organ transplants. This tool does not discriminate well between two similar individuals, but it performs

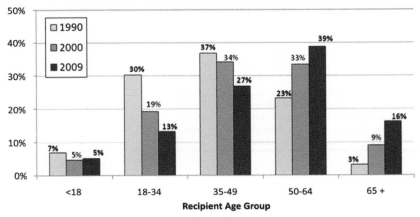

Fig. 5. Recipient age distribution for kidney transplants, United States, 1990, 2000, and 2009. (*Data from* Organ Procurement and Transplantation Network as of November 6, 2009.)

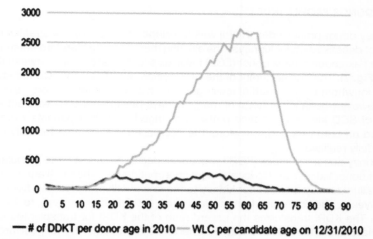

Fig. 6. Overall distribution of candidates and donors by age. DDKT, deceased donor kidney transplants; WLC, wait-list candidates. (*From* Ross LF, Parker W, Veatch RM, et al. Equal opportunity supplemented by fair innings: equity and efficiency in allocating deceased donor kidneys. Am J Transplant 2012;8:2115–24; with permission.)

well when dividing patients into broad categories. A lower estimated posttransplant survival (EPTS) score suggests longer posttransplant survival, and a higher score shorter survival. Examples of EPTS scores for various candidates are shown in **Table I.**

In the new allocation system, EPTS scores will be used to divide patients on the waiting list into the top 20% of scores and the remaining 80%. These 2 broad categories will be used to distribute kidneys with the longest potential survival to candidates with the longest estimated posttransplant survival, those in the top 20% of EPTS scores.

Table 1				
Estimated posttransplant survival vignettes: who is in the top 20%?				
Age (y)	**Dialysis Duration (y)**	**Diabetes**	**Prior Transplants**	**EPTS (%)**
18	0	No	No	1
25	0	No	No	1
18	2	No	No	2
25	5	No	No	5
25	2	No	Yes	7
40	0	No	No	8
18	0	Yes	No	12
25	0	Yes	No	12
40	5	No	No	17
50	0	No	No	18

Based on kidney wait-list registrations as of May 31, 2012. Data prepared by UNOS for the OPTN Kidney Transplantation Committee, October 2012.
Abbreviation: EPTS, estimated posttransplant survival score.

KIDNEY DONOR PROFILE INDEX

The kidney donor profile index (KDPI) was developed to improve risk stratification for survival of deceased donor kidneys. The existing method using standard criteria donor (SCD) and extended criteria donor (ECD) involves substantial overlap between the two groups (**Fig. 7**). The original intent of the ECD system was to list for ECD kidneys only patients for whom the trade-off of lower graft survival was offset by more rapid transplant. However, because survival of many kidneys designated ECD was better than survival of SCD kidneys, practice patterns changed such that patients were being registered on both lists and, therefore, the decreased waiting time for ECD kidneys was not fully realized.

The kidney donor risk index (KDRI) was developed to provide a more granular index of risk for donor kidneys and to locate them on a continuum.[7] The KDRI adjusts the risk of graft failure for any given donor kidney to the rate of failure for kidneys from donors aged 40 years. The scale runs from a relative risk of 0.5 (better survival), to 4.2 (worse survival). The KDPI transforms the hazard ratio of the KDRI for transplanted kidneys into a linear scale from 0% to 100%, where 0% represents the longest projected survival and 100% the shortest (**Fig. 8**).

KDPI variables:
- Donor age
- Donor height
- Donor weight
- Donor ethnicity
- History of hypertension
- History of diabetes
- Cause of death
- Serum creatinine
- Hepatitis C virus status
- Donation after circulatory death status

THE PROPOSED SYSTEM

The proposed allocation system will allocate kidneys in 4 sequences. The projected longevity of the kidney as determined by the KDPI will determine which sequence is

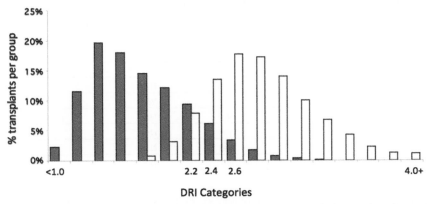

Fig. 7. Overlap of standard criteria and extended criteria donor kidneys. DRI, donor risk index.

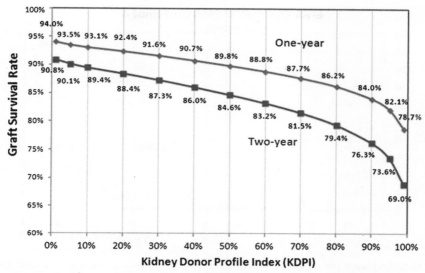

Fig. 8. Estimated graft survival rates by kidney donor profile index. (Source: OPTN.)

initiated. Stratification within the different sequences will be based on several factors used in the current system, primarily waiting time with contributions from HLA-DR matching and points for level of antibody sensitization. This factor was chosen because it is widely accepted by patients and it grounds this allocation system in the ethical principle of equity. Waiting time will be calculated either from time of listing with estimated glomerular filtration rate or creatinine clearance less than 20 mL/min, or from time of dialysis initiation (if dialysis was initiated before listing).

In the current allocation system, sensitized patients, as defined by calculated panel-reactive antibody (CPRA) greater than 80%, receive an additional 4 points on their allocation scores (roughly equivalent to 4 years of waiting time depending on geographic location). Work done by the OPTN Histocompatibility Committee demonstrated that this approach does not reflect the biology of the sensitized population, and that additional points should be awarded to sensitized patients on a continuous sliding scale (**Fig. 9**). Modeling suggests that this approach will help improve kidney offer rates for candidates with the highest degrees of sensitization, 98% to 100%.

In the new allocation system, as in the current one, all previous living organ donors, of kidneys and of other organs, receive priority for kidney transplant should they ever develop ESRD. This priority applies to first and subsequent transplants. In addition, points will be assigned based on HLA-DR matching, as this helps improve long-term survival without adversely affecting access to kidney transplant in minority populations. Also, in an effort to improve access for minority populations, kidneys from donors with blood type non-A1 (A2) and non-A1B (A2B) will be allocated to recipients in blood group B. Modeling suggests that this results in improved transplant rates for blood group B candidates proportional to their numbers on the waiting list.

Finally, in the new allocation system the ECD program is revised such that only waiting time is used to rank order candidates. ECDs are currently defined as all donors older than 60 years or older than 50 years with 2 of the following: hypertension, death from cerebrovascular accident, or serum creatinine level higher than 1.5 mg/dL. Under the new system, ECDs will be defined as all donors with KDPI greater than 85. This

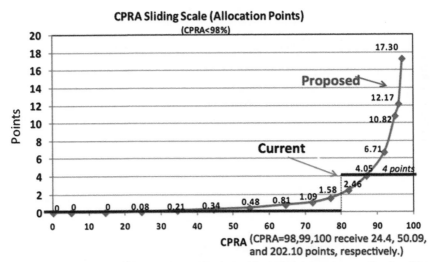

Fig. 9. Sliding scale for allocation points by calculated panel-reactive antibodies (CPRA). (Source: OPTN. Prepared for the Kidney Transplantation Committee, 2011.)

approach should make the timing of the organ offer more predictable and thus allow transplant centers to perform list maintenance in the patient group at most risk. In addition, organs will be offered at the regional level, bypassing local allocation, in an effort to expedite placement and perhaps encourage increased recovery of these organs.

Sequence A: Top 20% KDPI Kidneys to Top 20% EPTS Candidates

In this sequence, the top 20% of kidneys (those with the greatest predicted longevity) will be allocated to candidates in the top 20% of EPTS. Modeling suggests that in all donation service areas, the number of potential recipients in the top 20% of EPTS greatly exceeds the number of donor kidneys in the top 20% of KDPI (based on the large mismatch between supply and demand), so that projected waiting time is less than waiting time for candidates in the remaining 80% but still substantial. Therefore, it is not anticipated that candidates in the top 20% of EPTS will forgo living-donor kidney transplant in anticipation of receiving a deceased donor kidney of longer anticipated survival in a timely fashion; this would be contrary to the experience of pediatric patients once they were given priority for all donors younger than 35 years, the "Share 35" rule. Following implementation of the Share 35 policy, the number of living-donor kidney transplants in pediatric candidates declined noticeably. This decline was presumably related to pediatric candidates being able to receive high-quality deceased donor organs with little or no waiting time.

Sequence B: Kidneys with KDPI Between 20% and 35%, Pediatric Candidates

In the current allocation system, pediatric candidates receive priority for donors younger than 35 years. In the new system, pediatric candidates will receive priority for all kidneys with KDPI less than 35%.

Sequence C: Kidneys with KDPI from 20% to 85%

This allocation sequence will pair kidneys with very good predicted longevity with candidates whose expected survival is good but not as long as the expected survival of candidates in the top 20% EPTS. For candidates in this sequence, EPTS will not be a factor in allocation. For candidates with EPTS greater than 20%, kidneys will be allocated based on points given for waiting time, HLA-DR matching, and CPRA.

Sequence D: Kidneys with KDPI Greater than 85%, Revamped ECD

Sequence D will be an opt-in system that will likely benefit older candidates or candidates for whom the benefit of decreased time to transplant offsets the risk of decreased graft longevity. Kidneys with KDPI greater than 85% will be allocated solely on the basis of time on the waiting list, and will be offered simultaneously to the local area and the region. This approach represents the first attempt to increase geographic sharing in kidney allocation.

CRITIQUE

Any allocation system that attempts to distribute a limited resource across a variety of interest groups will, by definition, be a list of compromises. Perhaps the biggest compromise in the development of this new kidney allocation system has been diminishing utility, decreasing the number of life-years gained, in an effort to preserve equity for recipients of all ages (**Table 2**).

Despite this reduction in overall utility, the new allocation system makes significant progress toward eliminating extreme mismatches between donor and recipient longevity. More importantly, modeling suggests that allocating kidneys with greater longevity to recipients expected to live the longest reduces the number of recipients listed for repeat transplant.[8] This tendency could potentially make more kidneys available for transplant by effectively reducing the size of the waiting list.

Another significant advance for kidney allocation is use of a metric of survival. Whereas the EPTS is not good at distinguishing between similar individuals, it is good at dividing potential recipients into 2 broad categories. Similarly, using the KDPI system of ranking donor kidneys is an improvement over the SCD/ECD approach, as it reduces the misclassification inherent in any binary labeling system applied to a continuum of quality. Finally, the new system uses a more scientific approach to highly sensitized patients that more closely follows the biology of compatibility matching. These 3 enhancements, based on actual data and not on perception, help lay the foundation for further improvement in the kidney allocation system because they provide metrics that are fixed and can be analyzed for further refinements to the system, in comparison with a stable baseline. This approach will allow for changes that advance the overall goal of a more balanced and fair system.

Table 2
Utility and equity in the new proposed kidney allocation system compared with previously considered strategies for allocation

	Matching Strategy				
	National Utility	Local Utility	Age + Longevity	Age	Longevity[a]
Gain in life-years from each year of transplant	34,026	25,794	15,223	14,044	8380
Proportion of transplants in recipients aged ≥50 y (%)	10	29	46	45	52

[a] Current proposal.

SUMMARY

The proposed system for allocating kidneys for transplant makes significant progress toward eliminating deficiencies in the current system. In the proposed approach, extreme mismatches in longevity are minimized, highly sensitized patients are given more equal access to transplant, and metrics are applied to assess patient survival and organ quality. Moreover, access to kidney transplant is preserved across the age spectrum. Finally, aspects of the program, such as regional sharing of high KDPI kidneys and fewer patients returning to the waiting list for repeat transplant, have the potential to increase the supply of available kidneys.

ACKNOWLEDGMENTS

The authors thank Nan Booth, MSW, MPH, ELS, of the Scientific Registry of Transplant Recipients, for manuscript editing.

REFERENCES

1. Wolfe RA, Ashby VB, Milford EL, et al. Comparison of mortality in all patients on dialysis, patients on dialysis awaiting transplantation, and recipients of a first cadaveric transplant. N Engl J Med 1999;341:1725–30.
2. Stratta P, Coppo R. Audit on quality of life of patients with chronic kidney disease on dialysis and after transplant. G Ital Nefrol 2008;25(Suppl 41):S45–57 [in Italian].
3. Park IH, Yoo HJ, Han DJ, et al. Changes in the quality of life before and after renal transplantation and comparison of the quality of life between kidney transplant recipients, dialysis patients, and normal controls. Transplant Proc 1996;28: 1937–8.
4. United States Congress House Committee on Ways and Means. Subcommittee on Health. National Organ Transplant Act: hearing before the Subcommittee on Health of the Committee on Ways and Means, House of Representatives, Ninety-eighth Congress, second session, on H.R. 4080. February 9, 1984. Washington, DC: U.S. G.P.O.; 1984.
5. McCormick TR. Principles of bioethics. University of Washington School of Medicine; 1998. Modified 2008. Available at: http://depts.washington.edu/bioethx/tools/princpl.html. Accessed April 29, 2013.
6. Health Resources and Services Administration/Organ Procurement and Transplantation Network Kidney Transplantation Committee. Concepts for kidney allocation. 2011. Available at: http://optn.transplant.hrsa.gov/SharedContentDocuments/KidneyConceptDocument.PDF. Accessed April 29, 2013.
7. Roa PS, Schaubel DE, Guidinger MK, et al. A comprehensive risk quantification score for deceased donor kidneys: the kidney donor risk index. Transplantation 2009;88:231–6.
8. Israni A, Gustafson S, Salkowski N, et al. New proposed national allocation policy for deceased donor kidneys in the US and its possible impact on patient outcomes [abstract]. Am J Transplant, in press. Available at: http://www.atcmeetingabstracts.com/.

Kidney Paired Donation and Its Potential Impact on Transplantation

Meredith J. Aull, PharmD, Sandip Kapur, MD*

KEYWORDS

- Paired donation • Living donor kidney transplantation • Kidney exchange
- Incompatible • Nondirected donor • Desensitization • Altruistic donor

KEY POINTS

- Kidney paired donation (KPD) is the most promising resource available to increase the number of organs available for kidney transplantation.
- Blood type incompatible, crossmatch incompatible, and even compatible donor/recipient pairs can benefit from transplantation facilitated by KPD.
- Desensitization therapy in combination with KPD is an important option for highly sensitized kidney transplant candidates.
- Despite ongoing controversial issues surrounding KPD, the transplant community has made great strides in developing innovative and equitable solutions.

INTRODUCTION: NATURE OF THE PROBLEM

As of March 15, 2013, more than 95,000 patients were on the United Network for Organ Sharing (UNOS) waiting list for a kidney transplant from a deceased donor.[1] Presumably, a vast majority of these patients have no potential living donors, or have willing but incompatible donors. Traditionally, blood type (ABO) or immunologic incompatibility has limited living donor kidney transplantation.

Based on blood type distributions in the United States, about 1 of every 3 potential living organ donors will be ABO incompatible with their intended recipient. Immunologic incompatibility occurs when transplant candidates are exposed to foreign (nonself) human leukocyte antigens (HLA) through blood transfusion, pregnancy, and/or prior transplantation. Exposure to foreign HLA leads many patients to develop anti-HLA antibodies, which cause reactivity against potential organ donors. Patients with a high

Division of Transplant Surgery, NewYork-Presbyterian/Weill Cornell Medical Center, 525 East 68th Street, Box 98, New York, NY 10065, USA
* Corresponding author.
E-mail address: sak2009@med.cornell.edu

Surg Clin N Am 93 (2013) 1407–1421
http://dx.doi.org/10.1016/j.suc.2013.09.001
0039-6109/13/$ – see front matter © 2013 Elsevier Inc. All rights reserved.

surgical.theclinics.com

degree of sensitization (ie, a high antibody load) often have great difficulty in finding an organ donor to whom they will not have a significant immunologic reaction, which could lead to early and severe rejection of the allograft if transplantation were to occur. According to the 2011 Organ Procurement and Transplantation and Scientific Registry of Transplant Recipients annual data report, approximately 40% of adult patients waiting for a kidney transplant have some degree of sensitization, and about 10% are considered highly sensitized (defined as a panel-reactive antibody level >80%).[2]

Patients may be successfully transplanted using ABO-incompatible donors or by transplanting across a positive crossmatch[3,4]; however, these methods are not an ideal solution for patients with incompatible donors. Both methods require "desensitization," which is the use of pretreatments such as plasmapheresis, intravenous immunoglobulin (IVIG), rituximab, splenectomy, and/or mycophenolate mofetil to reduce anti-ABO (anti-A or anti-B) or anti-HLA titers to enable transplantation between the incompatible donor and recipient. However, the excess immunosuppression, morbidity (via increased risk of antibody-mediated rejection [ABMR] and its associated treatment), and cost associated with such transplants leave significant room for alternative solutions.[5,6] A meeting report from a symposium organized by the Roche Organ Transplantation Research Foundation agreed that because of the negative consequences of ABMR on the transplant allograft, the goal of the transplant community should be to prevent ABMR rather than treat it once it occurs.[6]

KIDNEY PAIRED DONATION: A SOLUTION TO THE SHORTAGE OF ORGANS FOR TRANSPLANT?

Paired exchange, as a mechanism to facilitate living donor kidney transplantation, is a concept first introduced by Rapaport[7] in 1986 as a solution to the shortage of deceased donor organs. Rapaport proposed an international registry whereby eligible and willing but ABO-incompatible living donors could donate via exchange facilitated through this registry. Donors would undergo simultaneous nephrectomy, transport of the donated organs would occur via courier, and implantation into the recipients would occur simultaneously.

Nearly 2 decades after the concept was first introduced, paired exchange came to be a somewhat routine occurrence at a few transplant centers,[8,9] although the logistical issues associated with international exchanges have not yet been solved. National exchange programs have been successfully developed in South Korea,[8] the Netherlands,[9] and the United States.[10,11] However, the concept has evolved from simple exchanges between 2 incompatible donor/recipient pairs to complex chains consisting of up to 30 pairs.[12] Proceedings from a 2012 consensus conference describe KPD as an "elegant but complex solution" to the shortage of organs available for transplant.[13] As seen in **Fig. 1**, paired donation has facilitated an increasing percentage of living donor kidney transplants in the United States over the past decade.[1]

KIDNEY PAIRED DONATION MODELS

As already described, the initial concept proposed by Rapaport has rapidly evolved into much more complex exchanges. The types of exchanges are described herein and are illustrated, in ascending order of complexity, in **Fig. 2**.

Kidney Exchange

As initially described by Rapaport, kidney exchange occurred between 2 donor/recipient pairs who were incompatible and, through participation in a registry, were

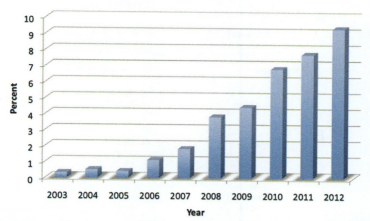

Fig. 1. Percentage of living donor transplants from paired donation in the United States.

matched with each other to create ABO-compatible transplants (see **Fig. 2**A). This process has been described as a "conventional" exchange.[14]

Expansion of the initial concept occurred by allowing both ABO-incompatible and immunologically (crossmatch) incompatible pairs to participate (see **Fig. 2**B), thus expanding the patient population that could be helped by donor exchange. This concept has been described as an "unconventional" exchange.[14]

In 2005, Montgomery and colleagues[14] from Johns Hopkins first reported their single-center experience using 10 paired donations to facilitate 22 kidney transplants, using a combination of both conventional and unconventional exchanges. For each paired donation, operations were performed simultaneously, and anonymity was maintained until after the surgeries. Being a referral center for difficult transplants (owing to experience with ABO-incompatible and positive crossmatch transplants), the Hopkins experience was particularly notable for its success in transplanting despite a pool of candidates who were difficult to match.

List Exchange

List exchange (see **Fig. 2**C) allows the incompatible donor of a donor/recipient pair to donate his or her kidney to the deceased donor waiting list, and in exchange the intended recipient receives priority on the deceased donor waiting list. Critics of this model point out that the majority of pairs participating in such an exchange will be ABO incompatible with an ABO non-O donor and an ABO O recipient, which is unfair to the ABO O recipients on the waiting list who will have to wait longer for an ABO O deceased donor kidney.

In 2004, representatives from transplant centers in UNOS Region 1 (New England) reported on implementation of a living donor/list exchange program, which had facilitated 17 transplants by the end of 2003.[15]

Domino Paired Donation

The domino paired donation (DPD) model (also referred to as a "closed" chain) begins with donation by a nondirected donor (NDD), also known as altruistic or Good Samaritan donor (see **Fig. 2**D). NDDs are living kidney donors who come forward to donate despite not having an intended recipient for their kidney. The first reported kidney donation by an NDD in the United States was in August 1999.[16] By representing the

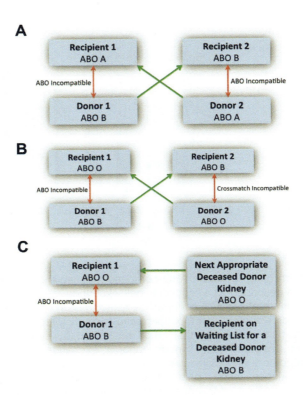

Fig. 2. (*A*) "Conventional" kidney exchange. Recipient/Donor Pair 1 and Recipient/Donor Pair 2 are both blood type (ABO) incompatible. By exchanging donors through KPD, Recipient 1 will receive a kidney from Donor 2, while Recipient 2 receives a kidney from Donor 1. (*B*) "Unconventional" kidney exchange. Recipient/Donor Pair 1 are blood type (ABO) incompatible while Recipient/Donor Pair 2 are ABO compatible, but a positive crossmatch prevents the donation. By exchanging donors through KPD, Recipient 1 will receive a kidney from Donor 2, while Recipient 2 receives a kidney from Donor 1. (*C*) List exchange. Recipient/Donor Pair 1 are blood type (ABO) incompatible. In list exchange, the incompatible living donor donates a kidney to a patient on the waiting list for a deceased donor kidney. Then the original intended recipient receives priority for the next appropriate deceased donor kidney. (*D*) Domino paired donation. Recipient/Donor Pairs 1 and 3 are blood type (ABO) incompatible while Recipient/Donor Pair 2 is crossmatch incompatible. In domino paired donation, a nondirected (altruistic) donor begins a chain of transplants by donating to Recipient 1; Recipient 1's Donor (1) then donates to Recipient 2, Recipient 2's Donor (2) donates to Recipient 3, and Recipient 3's Donor (3) donates a kidney to a patient on the waiting list for a deceased donor kidney; the chain then ends. (*E*) Nonsimultaneous extended altruistic donation (NEAD). Recipient/Donor Pairs 1 and 3 are blood type (ABO) incompatible, while Recipient/Donor Pair 2 is crossmatch incompatible. In domino paired donation, a nondirected (altruistic) donor begins a chain of transplants by donating to Recipient 1; Recipient 1's Donor (1) then donates to Recipient 2, Recipient 2's Donor (2) donates to Recipient 3, and Recipient 3's Donor (3) then waits to donate until a suitable match is found within the KPD registry, and the chain continues at that time. Donor 3 is considered a "bridge" donor, and the donor's role in kicking off the continuation of the chain mimics that of the initial nondirected donor.

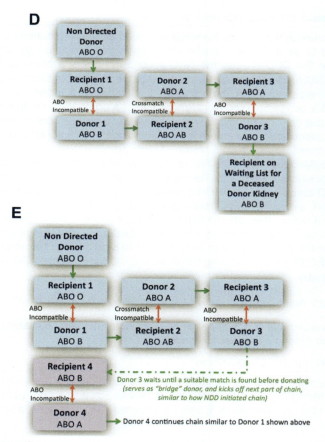

Fig. 2. (*continued*)

general population, these NDDs present an important source of ABO O donors. This initial donation starts a "chain" of transplants whereby the NDD kidney recipient's intended but incompatible donor is matched to a compatible recipient, then that recipient's intended but incompatible donor is matched with a compatible recipient, and so on. If a compatible recipient cannot be found for the last donor's kidney within the KPD registry, the kidney is allocated to the deceased donor waiting list according to UNOS policy, and the chain ends (thus the term "closed" chain).

After successfully implementing KPD in the mid-1990s, the Korean KPD program began using DPD in 2001, and performed 179 transplants as a result between 2001 and 2007.[17] Seventy chains (the majority of which transplanted 2 or 3 patients) were initiated by an altruistic donor, and the last kidney went to a patient without a living donor. Donors traveled to the recipient transplant center, and operations were not simultaneous, but did occur within a short time frame (goal <7 days). In the United States, Montgomery and colleagues[18] first proposed the use of NDDs to generate multiple transplants via DPD in 2006. Roth and colleagues[19] performed simulations showing that the use of NDDs to start chains of transplants in the DPD model could increase the number of kidneys available for transplant.

Nonsimultaneous Extended Altruistic Donation

A transplant chain in the nonsimultaneous extended altruistic donation (NEAD) model (also referred to as an "open" chain) also begins with donation by an NDD (see **Fig. 2**E). Like the DPD model, the NDD's donation starts a chain of transplants whereby the NDD kidney recipient's intended but incompatible donor is matched to a compatible recipient, then that recipient's intended but incompatible donor is matched with a compatible recipient, and so on. If a compatible recipient cannot be found for the last donor's kidney, the donor serves as a "bridge" donor who waits until a suitable recipient/donor pair enters the registry, and the chain continues on (thus the term "open" chain).

Rees and colleagues[10] were the first to report use of a NEAD chain, which facilitated 10 living donor kidney transplants. Their group combined several different techniques, including KPD combined with ABO-incompatible transplantation and combined with desensitization, as well as participation of a compatible pair.

The National Kidney Registry (NKR) has had great success in transplanting patients via NEAD chains.[11] The NKR model combines NEAD and DPD; bridge donor characteristics guide the decision for that bridge donor to start another transplant chain (for example, if ABO O) versus donating to the waiting list (for example, ABO AB or unable to wait to donate).

ACTIVE KIDNEY PAIRED DONATION PROGRAMS IN NORTH AMERICA

There are several single and multicenter KPD registries actively facilitating transplants today in North America, as described here.

Multicenter KPD in the United States

There are currently 7 multicenter KPD programs functioning in the United States,[13] providing a driving force for competition and innovation among programs (**Table 1**). Despite the individual successes of these multicenter KPD programs, a single national

Table 1
Multicenter KPD programs, United States

KPD Program	Transplants Facilitated[a]	Web Site
Alliance for Paired Donation	22 (between 7/18/07 and unknown/2010)[20]	http://www.paireddonation.org
Johns Hopkins	45 (between 2001 and 8/27/07)[21]	http://www.hopkinsmedicine.org/transplant/programs/kidney/incompatible/paired_kidney_exchange.html
National Kidney Registry	677 (between 2/14/2008 and 3/28/2013)[22]	http://www.kidneyregistry.org
North American Paired Donation Network	Not available	http://www.paireddonationnetwork.org
North Central Donor Exchange Cooperative	Not available	http://www.ncdec.org
United Network for Organ Sharing	19 (between 10/2010 and 3/2012)[23]	http://optn.transplant.hrsa.gov/resources/KPDPP.asp
Washington Regional Transplant Community	Not available	http://www.beadonor.org

[a] Transplants facilitated derived from published literature or publicly available sources.

KPD program is the ultimate goal, as it would generate the largest pool of donor/recipient pairs and thus could facilitate more transplants. Compared with geographically smaller countries with a small number of transplant centers (such as the Netherlands and Korea), implementation of a national KPD program in the United States is understandably more challenging because of its size and more than 225 kidney transplant programs.[1]

Single-Center KPD in the United States

The kidney transplant program at Methodist San Antonio has been the most successful single-center KPD program in the United States, having performed 134 kidney transplants over approximately 3 years.[24] This program includes incompatible donor/recipient pairs as well as compatible pairs with an age discrepancy, and utilizes the database developed at Johns Hopkins for the purpose of matching donors and recipients for KPD. This program attributes its success (despite being a single center with a limited pool) to prospective education of donor/recipient pairs about KPD, comprehensive immunologic profiling of donor and recipient, flexible assignment of unacceptable antigens, storage of blood samples for future testing, use of desensitization, subtyping of ABO A donors, and inclusion of compatible pairs.

Multicenter KPD in Canada

In Canada, the Living Donor Paired Exchange (LDPE) kidney transplant registry is a partnership between Canadian Blood Services and transplant programs across the country, designed to facilitate living kidney donations between patients with a willing but incompatible donor and other pairs in the same situation. The program, initially launched as a pilot program in 3 Canadian provinces in 2009, had performed 171 kidney transplants by October 2012.[25]

CLINICAL OUTCOMES

Experience with KPD to date shows that transplants facilitated by KPD have outcomes equivalent to those of traditional living donor kidney transplantation.[11,14,21,26] These excellent outcomes are particularly impressive considering the extent of sensitization shown by many recipients in the registry pool.

WHAT FACTORS HAVE DRIVEN THE INCREASE IN PAIRED DONATION–FACILITATED TRANSPLANTS?
Keys to Success

Participation of nondirected donors

It is through the participation of NDDs that KPD programs have had greater success in facilitating transplants in recent years. By introducing a donor to the KPD pool who has no linked recipient, the pool of donors increases and mimics the characteristics of the general population, bringing much-needed ABO O donors into the pool. A recent analysis shows that use of NDDs for transplant chains has the ability to significantly amplify the benefit provided by NDDs, because each NDD generates an average of 5 transplants, or even more if the donor is ABO O.[27] Most KPD programs require psychiatric evaluation as part of the evaluation process for potential NDDs.

Large pool size

By having a large pool of incompatible donor/recipient pairs, there is an increased chance of finding an acceptable match. A large pool generally also increases the heterogeneity of the pool, which is beneficial in matching donors with recipients. In conjunction with the advanced software used by successful KPD programs, a larger pool can generate many more potential matches for incompatible pairs.[28]

Mathematical modeling software/matching algorithm

Many mathematical models have been developed to identify matches for the donor/recipient pairs participating in KPD registries. These models vary greatly in terms of the factors used in the model, although most use similar criteria for determining matches. The frequency at which "match runs" occur also varies greatly among KPD programs.

The common factors include:

- Donor and recipient ABO type
- Virtual crossmatch results using donor HLA antigen and recipient anti-HLA antibody profile
- Preferences related to donor travel (ie, distance willing to travel)
- Waiting time within KPD registry
- Limiting ABO O donors from donating to ABO non-O recipients
- Entering ABO A2 donors as ABO O* donors[29]

As more advanced software has been developed to facilitate KPD, there has been movement away from the traditional integer-programming algorithms used in early models. The NKR software is built on technology utilizing concepts from capital market exchange systems.[28] An outcome-based strategy for generating matches within KPD as a method to improve both the quantity and quality of transplants has also been proposed.[30]

Much research has focused on the ability of the 2 newest KPD models (DPD and NEAD) to generate the highest numbers of transplants. However, there does not yet seem to be a definitive answer, owing to the numerous factors involved in the modeling process.[31,32]

Virtual crossmatch

The availability of advanced tools from immunology has been instrumental in the growth of KPD. Traditionally, a crossmatch is performed by using serum from both the potential organ donor and transplant candidate, and use of the complement-dependent cytotoxicity test and flow cytometry to detect antibodies that react with donor HLA antigens. A virtual crossmatch utilizes identified donor-specific antibody titers/unacceptable antigens for a particular candidate (via screening with single antigen beads such as Luminex) and the detailed HLA typing of the potential donor to assess for potential reactivity. Virtual crossmatching is successfully used by several large KPD registries,[33,34] reducing logistical issues and costs associated with performing a traditional crossmatch. Traditional crossmatch testing is then performed between matched donor/recipient pairs to assess compatibility before transplantation.

Flexible assignment of unacceptable antigens may be important,[24,35] particularly when attempting to identify potential donors for highly sensitized transplant candidates. By not excluding antigens to which the candidate has a low level of antibody, a KPD registry can increase the pool of potential donors for that recipient; this is where willingness to use a combination of KPD and desensitization can increase success in identifying a suitable donor.

Willingness to combine KPD with desensitization protocols

Montgomery and colleagues[35] have described success with a "hybrid" model that uses KPD to identify a more immunologically favorable donor (although not completely free of potential reactivity) and then use desensitization techniques to facilitate transplantation. This method enables use of less immunosuppression for desensitization, and an increased chance of successful transplantation. This option is of great importance given that highly sensitized recipients (panel-reactive antibody >80%) have had low match rates (<15%) in KPD experience to date.[35] Sharif[36] reports another strategy successfully used by the Hopkins transplant program, termed "rescue KPD". Patients unsuccessfully desensitized against their donor are reprofiled for anti-HLA antibody after the desensitization therapy, and the incompatible pair is then entered into the KPD program.

Transplant center dedication of resources to KPD program

The complexity of today's KPD exchanges requires participating transplant centers to allocate dedicated staff to their KPD program. KPD transplants are logistically challenging, and centers wishing to participate have to give thought to the infrastructure and resources needed for meaningful participation. Coordination and logistical support throughout the process is essential. Flexibility in scheduling of both donor and recipient cases is desirable, as there may be a need to reschedule or rearrange at short notice to ensure continuity of the transplant chains.

Active participation and support from hospital administration and finance are essential, as complex insurance and financial issues may arise. A clear understanding of the benefits of transplantation over dialysis and the positive financial impact of a successful living donor transplant by hospital administrators is essential.

It has been suggested that transplant programs considering joining a KPD registry should identify a KPD Champion to lead their program, and that each KPD registry should identify mentors who have successfully implemented KPD at their own center, to provide guidance and support to new transplant centers.[13] A KPD Champion is essential in bringing together key players from both the transplant program and administration.

A transplant coordinator with hands-on experience is needed to manage the complex logistics of KPD, including entry of donors and recipients into the registry, receiving match offers, and managing logistics among transplant centers involved in a particular chain. The coordinator also maintains medical records for donor organs procured at outside centers needed for the recipient medical record, tracks the organ(s) en route to the transplant center, fields issues arising on the day of the surgery, and arranges contact between donors and recipients who wish to meet after their surgeries.

ONGOING ETHICAL ISSUES AND CONTROVERSIES

As KPD has evolved and become more complex, several ethical debates have dominated discussions about the field. The reader is referred to Melcher and colleagues[13] and other ethics-related studies[37–40] for a thorough discussion of these controversial issues, which are summarized here along with the potential solutions that have been proposed in the literature.

Loss of Donor Ability to "Back Out"

Issue(s):
- Participation in a KPD program may cause a potential donor to feel like they can no longer "back out" of donation by using the reason of incompatibility.
Proposed Solution(s):
- Education of potential donors is essential; donors must be aware that they can stop the donation process at any time, even up to the time of the surgery. Donors should be encouraged to bring up any and all concerns with their donor team, and

should understand that the donor team is there to advocate for them and can provide alternative reasons why the donor cannot participate in KPD.
- Creation of standardized educational materials and informed-consent documents has been proposed.

Participation of Nondirected Donors

Issue(s):
- The evaluation process for NDDs should include a psychiatric evaluation.
- Allocation of NDDs should not be arbitrary.

Proposed Solution(s):
- All NDDs must undergo a psychiatric evaluation as a routine part of their workup.
- For living donor kidneys being allocated to the deceased donor waiting list, the UNOS algorithm for allocating deceased donor kidneys should be used to ensure fairness and equity.

Disadvantage to ABO O Recipients

Issue(s):
- Because ABO O donors are universal donors and can donate to any blood type recipient, it becomes difficult to find ABO O donors for ABO O recipients.
- ABO O candidates represent 52% of the patients on the deceased donor waiting list.[1]
- List exchange can harm ABO O wait-list candidates by prioritizing ABO O kidneys to candidates whose ABO non-O donors donated to the waiting list, thus prolonging the waiting time of those already on the waiting list for an ABO O kidney.

Proposed Solution(s):
- Limit ABO O to ABO non-O donations (except when using to facilitate transplant for a highly sensitized non-O recipient).
- Subtype ABO A donors into A1 and A2; categorize ABO A2 donors as ABO O* donors to expand the donor pool, because A2 donors are less likely to cause immunologic reactivity[29]; measure anti-A2 titers in recipients to assess for compatibility.
- Allow compatible donor/recipient pairs (ie, ABO O donor with ABO non-O recipient who have no immunologic incompatibility) to participate in KPD to expand the pool of ABO O donors. As demonstrated by Ratner and colleagues,[41] inclusion of compatible pairs can facilitate transplantation of recipients with incompatible living donors.

Reneging of Donor/Simultaneous Versus Nonsimultaneous Surgeries

Issue(s):
- In cases where nonsimultaneous operations occur, a donor could renege if waiting to donate, particularly when the original recipient has already been transplanted.
- The risk of reneging may increase the longer a donor waits for the registry to find a suitable recipient, especially since life circumstances may change.

Proposed Solution(s):
- Chains initiated by an NDD eases the risk because although their original recipient has already been transplanted, and reneging would break the chain of future transplants, the recipients further down in the chain will still have their donor available for construction of another chain of transplants.
- Chains can be repaired (no irreparable harm to future recipients).
- Perform simultaneous operations when feasible.

Travel of Donor Versus Donor's Kidney

Issue(s):
- Requiring donors to travel forces them to have surgery and recover away from their home and support system.
- Donor travel is costly and is an out-of-pocket expense that is not covered by recipient insurance.

Proposed Solution(s):
- There is now extensive experience with shipping living donor kidneys across the United States.[42]
- Loss of donated organs has not been an issue; global positioning system devices may be used.[28]
- There has been no significant impact of cold ischemia time on living donor kidney transplant outcomes to date.[42]
- Payors may consider coverage of donor travel.[13]

Donor and Organ Quality

Issue(s):
- Different donor selection standards at different transplant centers could lead to inequality.
- Recipient surgeon relies on donor surgeon at another institution to provide a transplantable organ without significant surgical damage.

Proposed Solution(s):
- Standardization of donor selection criteria across participating centers.
- Close communication between donor and recipient surgeons to relay clinically relevant information that will influence the recipient surgeon.

Participation of Compatible Donor/Recipient Pairs in Kidney Paired Donation

Issue(s):
- Inclusion of compatible pairs (ie, ABO O donor with ABO non-O recipient who are immunologically compatible) could facilitate transplantation by providing key ABO O donors to the pool.
- Education is key to success in facilitating this type of participation without causing undue stress on the compatible donor/recipient pair (ie, feelings of guilt if pair does not wish to participate in KPD).
- Transplant centers cannot ethically directly request that compatible pairs participate.

Proposed Solution(s):
- Consider participation of compatible pair only if the recipient will derive benefit from participation (ie, will receive a kidney from a younger donor or more immunologically compatible donor).
- Limit the amount of time that a compatible pair must wait (ie, set a time limit on amount of time the pair will await a match; go forward to transplant with original compatible donor if no match identified through registry within the designated time frame).
- Both the donor and recipient could derive psychological benefit from helping additional patients in need of a transplant.

Should Donors and Recipients Meet?

Issue(s):
- Matched donors and recipients allowed to meet before the transplant could renege (ie, one pair could be unhappy with the age of the matched donor).

- Posttransplant meeting could cause distress to one or more parties if the outcome in recipient (or donor) is poor.

Proposed Solution(s):

- Matched donor/recipient pairs should be kept anonymous throughout the pre-transplant process.
- After transplant, matched donor/recipient pairs should meet only if both parties consent to the meeting.
- All donor/recipient pairs entering KPD programs should be educated about potential risk for poor outcome and be reminded of the altruistic nature of their participation in KPD, regardless of outcome.

Payment Structure for KPD

Issue(s):

- At present, lack of standardization between transplant programs, states, and/or insurance companies for payment of organ-acquisition fees, transportation of donated kidneys, and other billing issues causes delays in both transplants and payments to involved transplant centers.

Proposed Solution(s):

- Nationwide standardization has been proposed through development of a standardized organ-acquisition charge to be used by all transplant centers involved in KPD.[43,44]

NEWYORK-PRESBYTERIAN/WEILL CORNELL EXPERIENCE WITH KPD THROUGH PARTICIPATION IN THE NATIONAL KIDNEY REGISTRY

The mission of our transplant program is to maximize opportunities for transplantation for all patients, and in the past 5 years KPD has become an important option for our patients. As a founding member transplant center of the NKR, the kidney transplant program at our center (NewYork-Presbyterian/Weill Cornell) has been participating in KPD since 2008. As of the first week of April 2013, participation in KPD as part of the NKR has enabled us to transplant 86 patients. We have previously published our initial experience with the first 50 KPD-facilitated transplants at our center.[26]

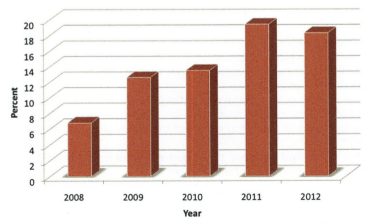

Fig. 3. Percentage of living donor transplants from paired donation at NewYork-Presbyterian/Weill Cornell Medical Center.

As seen in **Fig. 3**, KPD accounts for steadily increasing percentages of our living donor transplant volume, and in 2011 and 2012 accounted for almost 20% of our annual living donor kidney transplant volume.

The success of the NKR in facilitating KPD transplants is likely attributable to several factors. The NKR was started by a father familiar with the struggles of finding a compatible living donor for his daughter, and who approached the problem from a new and different perspective. In addition, collaboration among many of the major national kidney transplant programs, utilization of advanced software to match donors with recipients, and transparent policies and procedures followed by all participating transplant centers (publicly available at www.kidneyregistry.org) have contributed to the success of the NKR.

SUMMARY

KPD is an exciting and promising solution to the current shortage of organs available for kidney transplantation. By enabling kidney transplant candidates and their willing but incompatible donors to join a KPD registry with the goal of being matched up with other pairs, KPD facilitates an increase in living donor kidney transplantation. Benefits of living donor transplantation include outcomes superior to those of deceased donor kidney transplants and remaining a shorter time on the deceased donor waiting list. In addition to increasing the quantity of kidney transplants, KPD offers an improvement in quality, by increasing the numbers of living donor organs available to patients who might otherwise wait years on the deceased donor waiting list. KPD also provides a new opportunity for highly sensitized patients who might otherwise never receive a transplant. Movement toward one national KPD program and continued collaboration between currently participating centers may enable continued exponential growth of transplants facilitated through KPD, and offers a viable strategy to address the organ shortage in the United States.

REFERENCES

1. Available at: http://optn.transplant.hrsa.gov/data/. Accessed March 23, 2013.
2. Available at: http://srtr.transplant.hrsa.gov/annual_reports/2011/default.aspx. Accessed March 23, 2013.
3. Montgomery JR, Berger JC, Warren DS, et al. Outcomes of ABO-incompatible kidney transplantation in the United States. Transplantation 2012;93(6):603–9.
4. Vo AA, Petrozzino J, Yeung K, et al. Efficacy, outcomes, and cost-effectiveness of desensitization using IVIG and rituximab. Transplantation 2013;95(6):852–8.
5. Archdeacon P, Chan M, Neuland C, et al. Summary of FDA antibody-mediated rejection workshop. Am J Transplant 2011;11(5):896–906.
6. Bradley JA, Baldwin WM, Bingaman A, et al. Antibody-mediated rejection—an ounce of prevention is worth a pound of cure. Am J Transplant 2011;11(6): 1131–9.
7. Rapaport FT. The case for a living emotionally related international kidney donor exchange registry. Transplant Proc 1986;18(3 Suppl 2):5–9.
8. Park K, Moon JI, Kim SI, et al. Exchange donor program in kidney transplantation. Transplantation 1999;67(2):336–8.
9. de Klerk M, Witvliet MD, Haase-Kromwijk BJ, et al. Hurdles, barriers, and successes of a national living donor kidney exchange program. Transplantation 2008;86(12):1749–53.
10. Rees MA, Kopke JE, Pelletier RP, et al. A nonsimultaneous, extended, altruistic-donor chain. N Engl J Med 2009;360(11):1096–101.

11. Melcher ML, Leeser DB, Gritsch HA, et al. Chain transplantation: initial experience of a large multicenter program. Am J Transplant 2012;12(9):2429–36.

12. Available at: http://www.nytimes.com/2012/02/19/health/lives-forever-linked-through-kidney-transplant-chain-124.html?pagewanted=all&_r=0. Accessed March 28, 2013.

13. Melcher ML, Blosser CD, Baxter-Lowe LA, et al. Dynamic challenges inhibiting optimal adoption of kidney paired donation: findings of a consensus conference. Am J Transplant 2013;13(4):851–60. http://dx.doi.org/10.1111/ajt.12140.

14. Montgomery RA, Zachary AA, Ratner LE, et al. Clinical results from transplanting incompatible live kidney donor/recipient pairs using kidney paired donation. JAMA 2005;294(13):1655–63.

15. Delmonico FL, Morrissey PE, Lipkowitz GS, et al. Donor kidney exchanges. Am J Transplant 2004;4(10):1628–34.

16. Matas AJ, Garvey CA, Jacobs CL, et al. Nondirected donation of kidneys from living donors. N Engl J Med 2000;343(6):433–6.

17. Lee YJ, Lee SU, Chung SY, et al. Clinical outcomes of multicenter domino kidney paired donation. Am J Transplant 2009;9(10):2424–8.

18. Montgomery RA, Gentry SE, Marks WH, et al. Domino paired kidney donation: a strategy to make best use of live non-directed donation. Lancet 2006;368(9533): 419–21.

19. Roth AE, Sönmez T, Unver MU, et al. Utilizing list exchange and nondirected donation through 'chain' paired kidney donations. Am J Transplant 2006;6(11): 2694–705.

20. Rees MA, Bargnesi D, Samy K, et al. Altruistic donation through the Alliance for Paired Donation. Clin Transplant 2009;235–46.

21. Segev DL, Kucirka LM, Gentry SE, et al. Utilization and outcomes of kidney paired donation in the United States. Transplantation 2008;86(4):502–10.

22. Available at: www.kidneyregistry.org. Accessed March 28, 2013.

23. Available at: http://www.unos.org/docs/Update_MarchApril_12_KPD.pdf. Accessed March 28, 2013.

24. Bingaman AW, Wright FH Jr, Kapturczak M, et al. Single-center kidney paired donation: the Methodist San Antonio experience. Am J Transplant 2012;12(8): 2125–32.

25. Available at: http://www.organsandtissues.ca/s/english-public/living-kidney-donation/675-2. Accessed March 31, 2013.

26. Leeser DB, Aull MJ, Afaneh C, et al. Living donor kidney paired donation transplantation: experience as a founding member center of the National Kidney Registry. Clin Transplant 2012;26(3):E213–22.

27. Melcher ML, Veale JL, Javaid B, et al. Kidney transplant chains amplify benefit of nondirected donors. JAMA Surg 2013;148(2):165–9.

28. Veale J, Hil G. The National Kidney Registry: 213 transplants in three years. Clin Transplant 2010;333–44.

29. Hurst FP, Sajjad I, Elster EA, et al. Transplantation of A2 kidneys into B and O recipients leads to reduction in waiting time: USRDS experience. Transplantation 2010;89(11):1396–402.

30. Chen Y, Li Y, Kalbfleisch JD, et al. Graph-based optimization algorithm and software on kidney exchanges. IEEE Trans Biomed Eng 2012;59(7):1985–91.

31. Ashlagi I, Gilchrist DS, Roth AE, et al. Nonsimultaneous chains and dominos in kidney-paired donation—revisited. Am J Transplant 2011;11(5):984–94.

32. Gentry SE, Montgomery RA, Swihart BJ, et al. The roles of dominos and nonsimultaneous chains in kidney paired donation. Am J Transplant 2009;9(6):1330–6.

33. Ferrari P, Fidler S, Holdsworth R, et al. High transplant rates of highly sensitized recipients with virtual crossmatching in kidney paired donation. Transplantation 2012;94(7):744–9.
34. Cecka JM, Kucheryavaya AY, Reinsmoen NL, et al. Calculated PRA: initial results show benefits for sensitized patients and a reduction in positive crossmatches. Am J Transplant 2011;11(4):719–24.
35. Montgomery RA, Lonze BE, Jackson AM. Using donor exchange paradigms with desensitization to enhance transplant rates among highly sensitized patients. Curr Opin Organ Transplant 2011;16(4):439–43.
36. Sharif A, Zachary AA, Hiller J, et al. Rescue kidney paired donation as emergency salvage for failed desensitization. Transplantation 2012;93(7):e27–9.
37. Patel SR, Chadha P, Papalois V. Expanding the live kidney donor pool: ethical considerations regarding altruistic donors, paired and pooled programs. Exp Clin Transplant 2011;9(3):181–6.
38. Ross LF, Rubin DT, Siegler M, et al. Ethics of a paired-kidney-exchange program. N Engl J Med 1997;336(24):1752–5.
39. Ross LF. The ethical limits in expanding living donor transplantation. Kennedy Inst Ethics J 2006;16(2):151–72.
40. Fortin MC. Is it ethical to invite compatible pairs to participate in exchange programmes? J Med Ethics 2013. [Epub ahead of print].
41. Ratner LE, Rana A, Ratner ER, et al. The altruistic unbalanced paired kidney exchange: proof of concept and survey of potential donor and recipient attitudes. Transplantation 2010;89(1):15–22.
42. Segev DL, Veale JL, Berger JC, et al. Transporting live donor kidneys for kidney paired donation: initial national results. Am J Transplant 2011;11(2):356–60.
43. Irwin FD, Bonagura AF, Crawford SW, et al. Kidney paired donation: a payer perspective. Am J Transplant 2012;12(6):1388–91.
44. Rees MA, Schnitzler MA, Zavala EY, et al. Call to develop a standard acquisition charge model for kidney paired donation. Am J Transplant 2012;12(6):1392–7.

Management of Hepatocellular Carcinoma

Emad H. Asham, MD, FRCS[a],*, Ahmed Kaseb, MD[b],
R. Mark Ghobrial, MD, PhD, FRCS[c]

KEYWORDS

- Hepatocellular carcinoma (HCC) • Liver resection • Liver transplant
- Locoregional therapy • Systemic therapy

KEY POINTS

- Management of hepatocellular carcinoma (HCC) is a rapidly evolving field. In the past decade, with advances in liver surgery and transplant, curative treatment can now be offered to patients with HCC in compensated livers who are diagnosed early or to those who are within transplant criteria.
- Explanted livers have provided a growing understanding of the underlying mechanisms in hepatocarcinogenesis and diagnostic modalities.
- For those tumors not amenable to resection or transplantation, several locoregional therapies are available.
- For advanced tumors, molecular targeted therapies are yielding promising results.
- Because of the heterogeneity of the patients and the disease, many questions are still waiting for answers through well-designed, adequately powered, and bias-free multicenter, controlled, randomized trials.

INTRODUCTION

Management of hepatocellular carcinoma (HCC) is a challenging task because of the intricate underlying liver disease and the occult nature of the disease. Moreover, changing epidemiology and rapidly evolving diagnostic and therapeutic options add to the challenge. Because of the complexity of the disease, it requires a multidisciplinary approach involving hepatobiliary/liver transplant surgeons, hepatologists, oncologists, and interventional radiologists.

[a] Department of Surgery, Methodist J.C. Walter Jr. Transplant Center, Houston Methodist Hospital, Texas Medical Center, 6550 Fannin SM 1661, Houston, TX 77030, USA; [b] Department of Gastrointestinal Medical Oncology, The University of Texas MD Anderson Cancer Center, 1515 Holcombe Boulevard, Unit 426, Houston, TX 77030, USA; [c] Department of Surgery, Methodist J.C. Walter Jr. Transplant Center, Houston Methodist Hospital, Texas Medical Center, 6550 Fannin SM 1661, Houston, TX 77030, USA
* Corresponding author.
E-mail address: ehasham@houstonmethodist.org

Surg Clin N Am 93 (2013) 1423–1450
http://dx.doi.org/10.1016/j.suc.2013.08.008
0039-6109/13/$ – see front matter © 2013 Elsevier Inc. All rights reserved.
surgical.theclinics.com

EPIDEMIOLOGY

The incidence of HCC is increasing globally. HCC is the fifth leading cause of death from cancer worldwide in men and seventh in women.[1] Chronic hepatitis B virus (HBV) and hepatitis C virus (HCV) are responsible for 78% of cases of HCC globally. Epidemiology varies in different parts of the world. In the Unites States, the incidence of HCC has tripled in the past 2 decades.[2] HBV is the most prevalent risk factor for HCC in heavily populated sub-Saharan Africa and south east Asia. In Egypt, viral hepatitis is hyperendemic with the highest prevalence of HCV in the world at 10% to 20% of the general population. In the United States, the incidence of HCC is increasing at an alarming rate primarily caused by HCV and nonalcoholic steatohepatitis (NASH).[3,4]

RISK FACTORS

The most important risk factor for the development of HCC is a background of chronic liver disease, for example, liver cirrhosis, regardless of the cause. Hepatotropic viruses and excessive alcohol intake are the leading risk factors.

Viral Hepatitis

Viral hepatitis, both B and C, is transmitted via transfusion of blood and blood products, contaminated instruments during invasive procedures, intravenous injections, and sexual contact. Vertical transmission from mother to fetus can also lead to the disease. The chronicity of infection and progression to liver cirrhosis is oncogenic. A chronic hepatitis B state increases the incidence of HCC 20- to 100-fold more than noncarriers. This wide range is to the result of secondary factors that are associated with increased incidence of HCC including male gender, tobacco, alcohol, and coinfection with another hepatotropic virus such as hepatitis C and D. In HBV, HBx antigen plays a significant role in tumorigenesis by altering signal pathways. The HBx gene induces HCC in transgenic mice.[5] Amongst the many regions of the human genome that HBx interacts with is the tumor suppressor gene, p53.[6] HBV vaccine is the first vaccine that prevents cancer. In Taiwan, vaccination of newborns has reduced the incidence of HCC among Taiwanese children with a parallel decrease in the HBsAg carrier state and the incidence of HBV.[7]

HCV is the major underlying cause of HCC in Japan, the United States, and Egypt. Confounding factors are male gender, obesity, diabetes, iron overload, alcohol, tobacco, coinfection with HBV, and age. A meta-analysis of HCV interferon-based therapy, which included 4614 patients in 3 randomized and 15 nonrandomized trials, suggests that it could reduce the risk of development of HCC in responders.[8] There have been trials to develop a vaccine for HCV but the rapidly evolving mutations of the virus genome and the immunomodulation property of the virus make vaccine development a daunting task.

Hepatitis A and E are not implicated in the development of HCC.[9] Hepatitis D virus occurs as a coinfection with hepatitis B but its role in development of HCC is controversial.[10]

Natural history of viral hepatitis

Once infected with HCV, approximately 80% of patients progress to chronic hepatitis. About 20% of those develop cirrhosis. Once cirrhosis is established, the annual incidence of HCC is 3% to 8%. It takes about 30 years from the time of infection with HCV and about 10 years from the time of cirrhosis for HCC to develop.[11] During that time, the HCC evolves from molecular to preclinical to clinical phases. In HBV chronic infection, carcinogenesis may precede the development of cirrhosis.

Pathogenesis of HCC secondary to viral hepatitis

Liver cirrhosis, regardless of the underlying cause, encourages hepatocarcinogenesis. Both HBV and HCV are capable of causing acute infection that is clinically unapparent or progresses to persistent chronic infection. Chronic infection does not produce symptoms until later. Eventually fatigue, malaise, and other stigmata of chronic liver disease set in.

The liver is the primary site of viral replication and insult. HBV is a double-stranded DNA virus that replicates within the hepatocytes near the endoplasmic reticulum (ER). HCV is an RNA virus that, once uncoated within the hepatocyte cytoplasm, replicates using hepatocyte nuclear DNA. These repeated cycles of hepatocyte necrosis and regeneration endorse tumor development. The accelerated cell turnover rate increases the probability of spontaneous mutations or DNA damage.[12] Also, as the virus replicates continuously using the host hepatocyte genome, quasi-species are produced as a result of error-prone replication. These quasi-species are persistent in the face of a robust host immune response, which may explain the mechanism of other diseases associated with HCV (eg, nephropathy). This process also makes it difficult to produce a vaccine for HCV. Considering the architecture of the liver, the cycle of chronic injury and repair produces regenerative nodules and fibrosis. Fibrogenesis is a product of stellate cell activation. Under normal circumstances, stellate cells are responsible for building the scaffolding on which hepatocytes develop. As hepatitis sets in, stellate cells are stimulated by inflammatory cytokines and cause excessive fibrosis. Fibrosis is a poor prognostic factor when staging liver disease.[13]

Hepatotropic viruses also have direct carcinogenicity. In patients with HBV, a significant number of HCCs arise in noncirrhotic livers. HBV integrates into the DNA of infected hepatocytes. This process may dysregulate the control mechanisms on the cell cycle by chromosomal instability, viral proteins, and alteration of the human genome and protooncogenes.[14] Many of the HCV proteins have been shown to interfere with metabolism and signal transduction in infected hepatocytes, which could contribute directly to hepatocyte transformation and carcinogenesis.[15]

Alcoholic (Laennec) Cirrhosis

Excessive intake of alcohol is a significant risk factor for HCC. There is a synergistic relationship between drinking alcohol (>60 g/d) and both HBV and HCV infection in increasing the risk of HCC by approximately 2-fold.[16] In decompensated alcohol-induced cirrhosis, the annual risk of HCC is 1%.[17]

Obesity and Diabetes

Epidemiologic studies have shown that obesity and diabetes mellitus are risk factors for HCC in nonalcoholic steatohepatitis (NASH). They are also the main cause of cryptogenic cirrhosis.[18] Hassan and colleagues[19] reported a synergistic effect between HCV, alcoholic liver disease, and diabetes, with 90% of patients having fatty liver disease (FLD).

FLD

FLD is a wide spectrum of liver disease that includes nonalcoholic FLD (NAFLD) and NASH. FLD is associated with obesity and diabetes. The initial insult is accumulation of fat in hepatocytes. The second insult that ignites the inflammation, steatohepatitis, leads to cirrhosis and oncogenesis. The cause of the second insult is not clear. It seems that cirrhosis is a precondition for HCC to develop in a background of FLD.[20] HCV genotype 3 is also associated with FLD. In NASH, 20% of patients progress to liver fibrosis or cirrhosis, whereas, in NAFLD, only 3% of patients develop fibrosis or cirrhosis.[21]

Iron Storage Disease

Hemochromatosis, iron overload, and the HFE mutations C282Y of H63D are associated with increased risk of HCC, about 200-fold compared with the normal population.[22] The incidence of HCC in hereditary hemochromatosis is 21%.

Biliary Disease

Primary sclerosing cholangitis and primary biliary cirrhosis are precursors of HCC.[23] In stage IV primary biliary cirrhosis, the relative risk of HCC in female patients is 1.5.[24]

Schistosomiasis

In a case-control study of Egyptian patients, *Schistosoma mansoni* increased the risk of HCC only in the presence of HCV, with an odds ratio of 10.3 (95% confidence interval [CI] 1.3–79.8).[25]

Venous Occlusive Disease

Budd-Chiari syndrome secondary to vena cava obstruction leads to an increase in hepatocyte turnover. This is manifested by nodular hepatic hyperplasia. The association of this syndrome with HCC is uncommon. There have been case reports of HCC in livers affected by Budd-Chiari syndrome.[26,27]

Liver Adenoma

The risk of malignant transformation in solitary and multiple liver adenomas is 10%. Multiple adenomas are typically seen in women on oral contraceptives and in type I glycogen storage disease.[28] Recent reports suggested an association between activated β-catenin and a higher risk of malignant transformation of adenomas to HCC.[29,30]

Aflatoxin

Aflatoxin is produced by the fungi *Aspergillus flavus* in poorly stored grains such as rice and corn and in nuts. In a meta-analysis of aflatoxin hepatocarcinogenesis, the population attributable risk of aflatoxin-related HCC was found to be 23%.[31]

Tobacco

Epidemiologic studies have shown that the association between tobacco smoking and increased incidence of HCC is independent of HBV or alcohol abuse.[32]

SURVEILLANCE

The aim of HCC surveillance is to improve outcomes and decrease mortality. Several studies ranging from observational cohort and case-control studies to nonrandomized trials have demonstrated the benefit of surveillance comprising early diagnosis, the prospect of receiving potentially curative treatment, and significant reduction in HCC mortality.[33]

Screening is the application of a validated diagnostic test for a population at risk; surveillance is the application of a screening test at regular intervals. Once the surveillance test yields abnormal results, enhanced follow-up is required, which includes a series of investigations to confirm or refute the diagnosis.

Predictive scores for the risk of development of HCC have been established in patients with chronic HBV. Wong and colleagues[34] proposed age, albumin, bilirubin, HBV DNA, and cirrhosis as independent risk factors.

In patients with cirrhotic HCV, the annual incidence of HCC is 2% to 8%.[35] Platelet count has been shown to be a surrogate marker for the risk of HCC. Once the platelet count is less than 100×10^9/L, the risk of HCC increases regardless of liver function.[36]

Patients with liver cirrhosis due to causes other than viral hepatitis warrant surveillance. HCC develops in alcoholic liver cirrhosis,[37] steatohepatitis,[38] stage 4 primary biliary cirrhosis where the risk is equal to that due to HCV,[39] and genetic hemochromatosis where the relative risk is around 20.[40]

Patients on the liver transplant waiting list for end-stage liver disease (ESLD) secondary to 1 of the causes listed above are also at risk. They should be under surveillance. Early diagnosis and treatment impedes tumor progression, reduces the dropout rate, and improves patient and graft survival.

Serum α-fetoprotein (AFP) and liver ultrasonography (US) are the most frequently used tests for screening. In 1 study, screening of 1125 patients with chronic viral hepatitis showed a sensitivity of 100% using both serum AFP at a threshold of more than 10 ng/mL together with US. The sensitivity of liver US alone was 87% and that of AFP alone was 75%.[41] However, it has a low specificity and sensitivity 25% to 65% at a cutoff of 20 ng/L.[42] Serum AFP can be nonspecific and it is increased during flares of active hepatitis. It is also not sensitive in the case of small tumors.[43]

Liver US is the recommended primary surveillance test for HCC. It has a sensitivity of 60% and a specificity of 85% to 90%.[44] Classically, HCC appears hypoechoic on US. It can also appear isochoric with a halo, hyperechoic, or with mixed echogenicity. Computed tomography (CT) scans and liver magnetic resonance imaging (MRI) are superior to US specially for detecting lesions smaller than 2 cm, but they are too expensive to be used for surveillance. Both are confirmatory tests or when the lesion cannot be adequately characterized by US.

Transient elastography is a US-based noninvasive measurement of liver stiffness. Elastography correlates well with the stage of liver fibrosis. It was used to assess the risk of HCC but is awaiting further refinement and validation.[45]

The current recommendation of the American Association for the Study of Liver Diseases (AASLD) is that patients at high risk of developing HCC should undergo surveillance at an interval of 6 months using US.[46]

DIAGNOSIS

The best results of treatment of HCC rely on early diagnosis. Once HCC is diagnosed on surveillance based on US, CT and/or MRI become necessary to confirm the diagnosis and stage the tumor. The ASSLD have developed an algorithm for the diagnosis of liver tumors found during surveillance (**Fig. 1**).[47]

The diagnosis of HCC relies heavily on specific imaging features of the tumor. AFP is not specific for HCC. It can be increased in intrahepatic cholangiocarcinoma, certain colorectal liver metastases, and gastric cancer.[48,49] AFP is also increased in ataxia telangectasia and hereditary tyrosinosis. AFP has 3 different glycoforms: AFP-L1, AFP-L2, and AFP-L3. AFP-L3 seems to be more specific for HCC and is detected in 35% of patients with HCC less than 2 cm in size.[50] Another serologic test is des-carboxyprothrombin (DCP) also known as prothrombin induced by vitamin K absence II (PIVKA II). It has been used more for diagnosis than surveillance of HCC.[51] According to the results of the HALT-C (Hepatitis C Antiviral Long-term

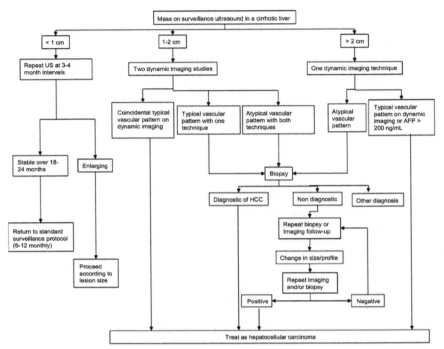

Fig. 1. Flowchart for management of hepatocellular carcinoma. (*From* Burix J, Sherman M. Management of hepatocellular carcinoma: an update. Hepatology 2011;53(3):1020–2; with permission.)

Treatment against Cirrhosis) study, DCP was found to be an inefficient test for HCC surveillance.[52] Serum proteomic profiling is a rapidly developing and promising new tool for the detection of HCC that seems more accurate than traditional biomarkers.[53]

US has a low sensitivity for lesions less than 1 cm and the detection of dysplastic liver nodules.[54] US contrast agents such as harmonic microbubbles improve the ability of US to diagnose liver lesions.[55] Dynamic contrast-enhanced CT reveals a highly specific imaging pattern of arterial enhancement followed by portal venous and delayed venous hypointensity, so-called washout.[56] On MRI, HCC appears hypointense, isointense, or hyperintense relative to the liver on T1-weighted images and hyperintense on T2-weighted images with intense enhancement on the arterial hepatic phase during a dynamic gadolinium contrast study.[57] MRI is superior to CT for delineation of suspicious hepatic nodules with an indeterminate enhancement pattern on CT.[58] Small lesions may be difficult to diagnose. Less suspicious lesions may be delineated by serial contrast-enhanced dynamic MRI.[59] However, clinical judgment, together with serologic markers and lesion biopsy, usually yields the diagnosis. The role of [18F]fluoro-2-deoxy-D-glucose (FDG)-positron emission tomography (PET) remains controversial due to its low sensitivity (50%–55%); HCC is inconsistent in accumulating FDG.[60]

The role of tumor biopsy in HCC is limited to lesions that cannot be safely characterized by the imaging modalities. The side effects of the procedure include hemorrhage and needle track seeding of 2%.[61]

STAGING

Once HCC is diagnosed, it has to be staged for prognosis and to plan the best available treatment. The plethora of staging systems for HCC reflects the heterogeneity and the complexity of the disease compounded by liver cirrhosis.

Several prognostic scoring systems have been developed based on clinical and laboratory data. The classic Child-Pugh score (**Table 1**) based on serum albumin, serum bilirubin, prothrombin time presented as the international normalized ratio (INR), the presence or absence of ascites and encephalopathy[62,63] remains reliable and reproducible to stratify the posthepatectomy risk of liver failure.

The Okuda score is based on tumor size in relation to the liver area, ascites, jaundice, and bilirubin level.[64] The model for end-stage liver disease (MELD) has been used to prioritize patients on the transplant waiting list. MELD is calculated as 0.957 × log_e(serum creatinine, mg/dL) + 0.378 × log_e(serum bilirubin, mg/dL) + 1.120log_e(INR) + 0.643.[65] It also predicts posthepatectomy liver failure. The Barcelona Clinic Liver Cancer Staging System (BCLC) (**Fig. 2**) has emerged as a scheme for treatment strategies including tumor ablation and liver transplant.[66] The cancer of the liver Italian program (CLIP) includes Child-Pugh class, tumor morphology, serum AFP, and portal vein thrombosis. Postresection or transplant staging systems that rely on the specimen pathology include the Japan integrated staging score (JIS) and the American Joint Committee on Cancer/International Union Against Cancer (AJCC/UICC) system. Wildi and colleagues[67] have outlined the details of the various staging systems in their critical review emphasizing the relative strengths and weaknesses of each.

CT of the chest, abdomen, and pelvis and a bone scan are essential to look for secondary disease and staging. The number of liver lesions, size including maximum diameter, location in the liver segments, vascular invasion, and any extrahepatic disease must be documented.

TREATMENT OPTIONS

Untreated HCC has a poor 5-year survival rate of 0% to 10%,[68] whereas HCC detected at an early stage has a 5-year survival rate of more than 50% after liver resection or liver transplantation. Nevertheless, most patients present at a late stage with poor liver function due to the insidious nature of the disease. Rapidly evolving treatment options are available for such patients (**Fig. 3**).

Table 1
Child-Pugh score for liver cirrhosis

Criteria	1 Point	2 Points	3 Points
Total bilirubin			
mg/dL	<2	2–3	>3
μmol/L	<34	34–50	>50
Serum albumin, g/L	>35	28–35	<28
International normalized ratio	<1.7	1.71–2.30	>2.30
Ascites	None	Mild	Moderate to severe
Encephalopathy	Absent	Grade I–II Responds to medication	Grade III–IV Refractory to medication

Class A: 5–6 points, class B: 7–9 points, class C: 10–15 points.

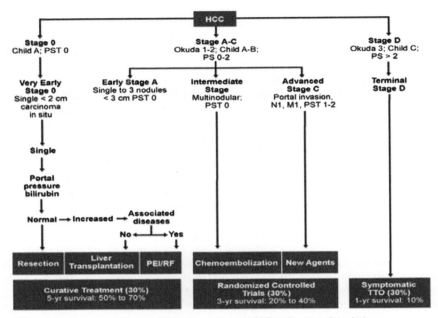

Fig. 2. The BCLC scheme for the management of HCC. (*From* Llovet JM, Bru C, Bruix J. Prognosis of hepatocellular carcinoma: the BCLC staging classification. Semin Liver Dis 1999;19:329–38; with permission.)

Liver Resection

Surgical resection is the best curative treatment of HCC, offering a 5-year survival rate of 60% to 70%.[69] However, only 10% to 15% of patients with HCC are candidates for liver resection.[70] The best candidates are those with a single lesion and well-preserved liver function. Contraindications include prohibitive cardiopulmonary status, nonresectable extrahepatic metastases, extensive bilobar disease, advanced cirrhosis, and close proximity to porta hepatis with involvement of hilar structures. The major causes of 30-day postoperative mortality is liver failure, hemorrhage, and sepsis.

Patients have to be evaluated carefully before resection to ensure that the future liver remnant (FLR) volume is capable of sustaining normal liver function and regenerating appropriately. Liver volumetric studies[71,72] and the iodocyanin green retention test at 15 minutes (ICG-R15)[73] have been the main methods for assessment of FLR volume and function, respectively. Normal livers tolerate resection up to 75% of parenchyma. Child-Pugh class A cirrhotic livers can tolerate resection up to 50% of liver parenchyma. However, not all Child-Pugh class A livers regenerate to the same capacity. Values of ICG-15R greater than 14% preclude resection. Tumors greater than 5 cm in diameter have a higher risk of recurrence and a worse prognosis, with a 5-year survival rate of 30%.[74] Other predictors of early recurrence are AFP level greater than 2000 ng/dL, nonanatomic resection, microvascular or macrovascular invasion, involved resection margins, and poorly differentiated tumors.[75] Preoperative thrombocytopenia ($<150 \times 10^3$ μL) is a prognostic marker for postoperative complications and liver insufficiency.[76]

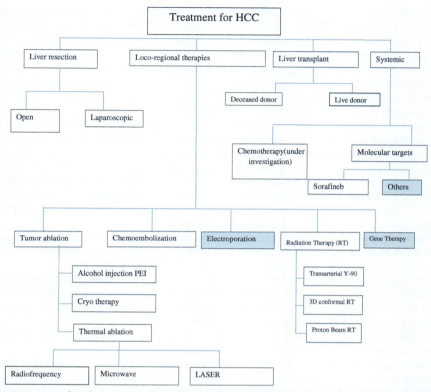

Fig. 3. Options for the treatment of HCC. Blue boxes are therapies still under investigation.

Portal vein embolization (PVE) has developed as a strategy for unresectable HCC secondary to small FLR volume. PVE was introduced by Makuuchi and colleagues[77] in 1982 to produce atrophy of the tumor-bearing lobe and hypertrophy of the contralateral remaining lobe. When liver volumetrics indicate that the FLR volume is inadequate, tumor ipsilateral PVE has been used to allow hypertrophy of the FLR, thus preventing posthepatectomy liver dysfunction.[78] PVE is indicated if the FLR is measured to be less than 40% of the preoperative liver volume with normal liver function. The procedure is achieved using 1 of 2 approaches: a transileocolic vein approach after a laparotomy and a more preferred percutaneous transhepatic approach in the interventional radiology suite. In the percutaneous transhepatic approach, the portal system is accessed by US-guided puncture of the transverse portion of the left portal vein. Gelatin sponges and steel coils have been used for embolization. FLR size increases from 19% to 36% of the total liver volume to 31% to 59%.[79] A standardized FLR of 20% or less or a degree of hypertrophy of less than 5% was found to be a prognostic factor for postoperative hepatic dysfunction.[80] However, cirrhotic livers may not increase in size adequately after PVE and the procedure is contraindicated in patients with moderate to severe liver dysfunction (ie, ICG-R15$\geq$20%). PVE leads to an increase in the ipsilateral hepatic artery flow[81] and may enhance tumor HCC growth, which is mainly supplied by hepatic artery branches. Sequential transarterial chemoembolization of the HCC 2 to 3 weeks before PVE suppresses the growth of the tumor.[82] In a meta-analysis of 75 publications, 85% of patients who received PVE underwent planned liver resections.[83]

Another strategy to induce hypertrophy of the contralateral liver lobe is stem cell therapy. Autologous CD34+ stem cells derived from the patient's bone marrow when mobilized in vivo and expanded in vitro then injected into the hepatic artery showed significant improvement in liver function and Child-Pugh score in alcoholic liver cirrhosis.[84] This pioneering work encouraged other researchers to take the concept further. In a report on 3 cases, intraportal administration of autologous bone marrow–derived CD133+ cells into the left lobe after segmental right PVE resulted in a 2.5-fold increase in the FLR volume.[85]

Preoperative measurement of the hepatic venous pressure gradient (HVPG) is gaining a lot of interest as a predictor of postoperative liver dysfunction. In a series of 39 patients who underwent liver resection for HCC, an HVPG of 5 mm Hg was found to be the cutoff for a significant increase in postoperative liver dysfunction, ascites, and longer hospital stay.[86] In another study, increased HVPG was associated with increased postoperative liver dysfunction when HVPG was greater than 7 mm Hg and increased 90-day mortality when HVPG was greater than 8 mm Hg, whereas classic indirect criteria (splenomegaly, esophageal varices, and thrombocytopenia) were not.[87]

The surgical armamentarium has expanded to include a variety of instruments such as the US scalpel, ultrasonic dissector, water jet dissector, radiofrequency, and staples, which allow safe liver resection with minimal blood loss.

Minimally invasive, laparoscopic liver resection has evolved to be safe for carefully selected Child-Pugh class A patients with a single peripheral lesion. The oncologic results are comparable with open surgery[88] with the benefit of less surgical trauma, shorter hospital stay, faster recovery, and better cosmetic surgical site. Using a laparoscopic bipolar radiofrequency device, liver resection was achieved with minimal intraoperative blood loss (48 ± 54 mL) and without blood transfusion.[89]

The development of liver transplantation surgical techniques, for example, total vascular exclusion, venovenous bypass, and ex vivo hepatic resection, has pushed the limits of liver resection. Tumors involving the inferior vena cava or major hepatic veins can be resected ex vivo followed by reimplantation of the liver with intent to cure.[90]

Moreover, computer-assisted and image-guided liver surgery is an emerging valuable tool that allows the transfer of two-dimensional (2D) images to three-dimensional (3D) images. 3D images with vascular and biliary mapping allow virtual resection and preoperative planning. Risk analysis using computer-assisted 3D images helps to alter resection planes and guide venous reconstruction to prevent venous outflow impedance.[91] The technology has been taken further and intraoperative image-guided surgery (IGS) is emerging to guide surgical instruments on preoperative planned CT scans. One clinical trial is evaluating the first generation of liver IGS.[92]

One of the main problems after liver resection with intent to cure is locoregional tumor recurrence, which occurs in 50% of patients within 3 years of resection or ablation.[93] Early recurrence within 2 years after resection is assumed to be due to residual occult disease, whereas late recurrence after 2 years is assumed to be de novo tumors.[68,75] Interferon therapy is believed to reduce recurrence and improve survival after R0 liver resection. In a meta-analysis of 7 randomized controlled studies evaluating 620 patients, interferon (6 studies used INF-α and 1 study INF-β) was shown to reduce the risk of recurrence with a pooled risk ratio of 0.86 (95% CI, 0.76–0.97). Nevertheless, 25% of patients had to undergo dose reduction or interruption of therapy because of side effects.[94]

Liver Transplantation

Orthotopic liver transplantation (OLT) offers the ultimate cure for both HCC and liver cirrhosis. The initial experience by Iwatzuki and colleagues[95] was marred with poor survival because of early recurrence. In the past decade, OLT has become the therapy of choice, when available, for a subset of HCCs not amenable to resection but within certain number and size criteria. The enthusiasm for OLT has been tampered by the shortage of deceased donor organs particularly in Asia. Such shortage led researchers to develop strict criteria to allocate scarce organs to selected HCC patients who can achieve survival comparable with nontumor patients. The Milan criteria were published in 1996 and include 1 HCC tumor of 5 cm or less in diameter or 3 tumors each 3 cm or less in diameter without vascular invasion on imaging or extrahepatic metastases. The 5-year and disease-free survival rates have been as high as 75% and 83%, respectively.[93] Enthused by the reproducibility of a 5-year survival rate of at least 70% at many centers, the criteria were expanded. The University of California San Francisco (UCSF) criteria include a single tumor 6.5 cm or less or 3 or fewer, the largest of which is 4.5 cm or less with a total diameter of 8 cm or less. The 1-year and 5-year survival rates were 90% and 75%, respectively.[96] Both popularized criteria consider the number and size of the tumor regardless of the tumor biology (eg, differentiation, molecular profiling). Current imaging modalities have a tendency to understage up to 10.4% and overstage up to 36.2% of HCC compared with explant pathology, as shown in the Eurotransplant review.[97] The University of Toronto developed a protocol for biopsy for large tumors up to 10 cm. Poorly differentiated tumors were excluded. Patients were treated aggressively before transplantation with ablative therapies. Survival in tumors beyond the Milan criteria was similar to those within the criteria.[98] After all, only 5% of patients with HCC are candidates for liver transplantation.[99] Advances in molecular biology have led to the development of tumor markers that correlate with prognosis and recurrence. These include categories such as proliferating indices, tumor promoter genes, tissue invasion and metastases markers, angiogenic markers, growth factors and genetic biomarkers, and micro-RNA. Most of the studies are retrospective and these markers are still awaiting studies comparing them to the scoring systems. Singhal and colleagues[100] offer a detailed review of such markers.

The Milan criteria were revisited by Mazzaferro and colleagues[101] in a multicenter data collection study incorporating 1556 patients. The "up to 7" criterion was reported to provide similar outcomes to the Milan criteria. Up to 7 means up to 7 tumors in number, the largest of which is less than 7 cm.

Locoregional ablative therapies introduced the concept of downsizing HCCs ineligible because of large size. In compensated livers, locoregional therapy can reduce the tumor to an acceptable size within conventional criteria. Posttransplant survival data are comparable in patients who underwent downsizing with those within conventional criteria.[102] Also, ablative therapies can offer bridging therapy for transplantation to decelerate tumor progression, minimize dropout, and improve posttransplant survival when the waiting interval is short. For example, transarterial chemoembolization (TACE) impedes tumor growth while patients are waiting for liver transplant.[103]

Once the HCC meets the transplantation criteria, the patient undergoes an extensive evaluation process for eligibility for transplantation.

There is no universal system for organ allocation. However, such systems should ensure prioritization according to the patient's clinical need, minimize waiting time and dropout, and administering justice between different patients groups. In the United States, acceptable deceased donor livers are allocated according to MELD score points. The United Network of Organ Sharing (UNOS) has adopted the Milan criteria since 2002 for listing HCC patients for transplantation. Tumors have to be at least 2 cm in diameter and patients are granted 22 exceptional points for the MELD score. These exception points are increased to 25 within 3 months should the patient be still waiting for OLT.[104]

Immunosuppression is the Achilles tendon of liver transplantation. It entails suscep-
tibility to infection, rejection, cost, compliance, and side effects. One of the most used
combinations is steroid, calcineurin inhibitors (CNIs), and mycophenolate mofetil
(MMF). CNIs, cyclosporine and tacrolimus, are potentially nephrotoxic and can induce
diabetes mellitus and hypertension. Drug levels have to be monitored frequently in
the early posttransplant period. Steroid sparing did not offer any advantage in HCV
recurrence after OLT although it reduced the incidence of diabetes.[105] Another immunosuppressant agent, mammalian target of rapamycin (mTOR or sirolimus), has antitumor and antiproliferative properties. A review of Scientific Register of Transplant
Recipients data on 2491 HCC patients showed survival benefit of sirolimus for patients
with HCC. Three-year and 5-year survival rates in sirolimus therapy groups were
85.6% and 83.1% compared with 79.2% and 68% in the nonsirolimus therapy group,
respectively (P<.05). In the same study, anti-CD25 (Campath, Zenapax, and Simulect)
induction therapy also demonstrated survival benefit.[106] On the other hand, in 1 multicenter study involving 412 patients, immunosuppression induction therapy with anti-
lymphocyte antibody (ATG) or anti-CD3 antibody (OKT3) was found to be a risk factor
for HCC recurrence after liver transplant.[107] These results emphasize the need for prospective, multicenter, randomized, controlled studies to solve this debate.

Living donor liver transplantation (LDLT) offers one solution to the ongoing shortage
of deceased donor organs. It eliminates the unpredictable waiting time and the risk of
dropout because of tumor progression while waiting. Living donors undergo extensive
evaluation including ethical, clinical, and psychological consideration. Donor safety is
the prime concern for transplant surgeons. In a series of 28 adult-to-adult LDLT for
HCC, the tumor recurrence rate was higher than with deceased donors, 28.6% versus
12.1%, respectively, with no difference in overall survival. Tumor poor differentiation
was a predictor for early recurrence.[108] The recurrence rate may be higher in LDLT
because HCCs with aggressive biology declare themselves while patients are on
the list awaiting deceased donor livers and then drop out.

Tumor Ablation

In the past decade, locoregional therapies for liver tumors have advanced remarkably
improving patient survival. These therapies can be applied under US or CT guidance
with local anesthesia, laparoscopically, or during open resection for contralateral lobe
small lesions.

Radiofrequency ablation

Very high frequency radio waves (450–500 kHz) generate localized intense heat
(50°C–100°C) that causes tissue coagulative necrosis. The high alternating current
generating the radio waves is delivered intratumorally via an electrode needle. The
size of the ablated area depends on the current intensity, the length and gauge of
the needle tip, and the duration of application. The maximum diameter of the tumor
should be equal to or less than 5 cm. Heat energy can be compromised by the cooling effect of the rich vascular supply of HCC and vicinity to large intrahepatic vessels
leading to incomplete ablation. In tumors 3 to 5 cm in diameter, radiofrequency ablation (RFA) produced complete tumor necrosis in 80% to 90% of treated HCC.[109]
Image-guided RFA can be applied percutaneously, laparoscopically, or via a laparotomy. In a series of 110 patients with cirrhotic livers, 149 HCC nodules were treated
with RFA and followed up for a median of 19 months. The local recurrence rate
was 3.6% and new liver lesions and extrahepatic metastases developed in
49.5%.[110] With recent advances in intraoperative US, it has become more sensitive
for detecting small tumors that are otherwise undetectable with other imaging

modalities. In addition, laparoscopic inspection of the liver and peritoneal cavity may provide more accurate staging.[111] However, this comes at an additional cost of general anesthesia and equipment. The complication rate of RFA is about 12% including liver abscess, subcapsular hematoma, intraperitoneal hemorrhage, hemobilia, biliary strictures, pneumothorax when done percutaneously, and liver failure.[112] Preoperative planning and careful consideration of the tumor location in relation to major hepatic vessels and bile ducts can minimize such complications. The confluence of the main bile ducts is vulnerable to thermal ablation applied to tumors at the bifurcation of the portal vein. Real-time US can assess the effectiveness of the ablation. Contrast-enhanced sonography helps to detect residual tumors and guide reapplication of the probes.[113] Follow-up CT scan is obtained after the peritumoral hyperemic rim has resolved, typically at 4 weeks, to assess the tumor ablation.

Advances in technology has taken RFA into new territory: intravascular ablation. Habib VesCoag is a monopolar/bipolar, radiofrequency, endovascular catheter designed to occlude blood vessels selectively. The catheter has a channel for delivery of chemotherapy as well. The initial experience in a cohort of 13 patients including 7 with HCC demonstrated safe angiographic target vessel occlusion in12 patients using monopolar endovascular RFA.[114]

Alcohol injection
Percutaneous injection of ethanol (PIE) into the tumor induces tumor necrosis by dehydration, protein denaturation, and vessel thrombosis. The injections are typically repeated at short intervals, weekly or biweekly, for up to 8 sessions. Tumors close to the liver capsule are contraindicated because of the risk of bleeding and intraperitoneal leakage, which can cause intense pain. The tumoricidal effect of PEI is about 70% in HCC less than 3 cm in diameter.[115] Tumors larger than 5 cm are not suitable for PEI. Although the low cost of PEI makes it an attractive HCC ablation modality, the results are inferior to RFA. In 1 prospective nonrandomized study, RFA achieved higher ablation rate on HCCs less than 3 cm than PEI (90% vs 80%) with fewer treatment sessions (12% vs 0%) albeit with more complications.[116]

Microwave
Microwave coagulation therapy (MCT) generates thermal energy at a frequency of 2450 ± 50 MHz, which causes cellular damage by protein coagulation at temperature greater than 50°C. The microwave dielectric heat is delivered via a needle electrode inserted into the tumor. MCT is restricted to tumors less than 2 to 3 cm to achieve complete tumor ablation.[117] As in RFA, MCT should be avoided in tumors near porta hepatis to avoid thermal injury to hilar structures. Complications of MCT are the same as for RFA. The local 1-year recurrence rate of HCC after MCT is 12.5%.[118]

Laser
Insertion of a neodymium-yttrium-aluminum-garnet (Nd-YAG) laser fiber can ablate HCC tumors up to 2 cm. Using multiple fibers can ablate larger tumors. The maximum diameter for adequate tissue ablation is 5 cm. In 1 series, complete tissue necrosis was accomplished in 82% of HCC nodules treated. However, cirrhotic patients have to be chosen carefully as liver failure and death have been reported in patients with Child C cirrhosis.[119]

Cryoablation
Cryotherapy has been used for the treatment of primarily metastatic liver tumors since the 1980s. Tissue ablation is achieved by freezing interstitial tissue fluid to subzero temperatures resulting in cellular dehydration and destruction of cellular structures.

Cryoprobes are cooled by liquid nitrogen or liquid argon. Probes are usually intro-duced during surgery using intraoperative US. The frozen tissue can be monitored in real time as a growing hyperechoic ice ball. Cryotherapy is most effective for tumors less than 5 cm. Major blood vessels adjacent to the tumor can cause a heat-sink ef-fect, reducing the freezing effect. Cryotherapy was found to be effective for treatment of unrespectable HCC.[120] Complications specific to cryotherapy include cracking of the liver parenchyma, freezing injury to adjacent structures, biloma, and biliary fistulas. The cryoshock phenomenon is a syndrome involving thrombocytopenia, dissemi-nated intravascular coagulopathy, adult respiratory distress syndrome, and acute renal failure and has been observed after cryoablation of large tumors.[121] Cryoablation has fallen out of favor in the past decade.

TACE

The rational of local chemoembolization is the dual blood supply of the liver. Although the parenchyma is primarily perfused with the portal blood supply, established HCC lesions are supplied by the hepatic artery, hence the rational of delivering the chemo-therapeutic agent via hepatic artery branches. Locally advanced tumors that are not amenable to surgical resection or transplantation are the main indication for TACE. TACE has also been used to downstage inoperable HCCs to offer the chance of cura-tive resection.[122] It has also been used for treatment of HCC while patients are on the transplant list for tumor control. Transarterial therapy can be either bland therapy, that is, only embolization of the tumor feeding vessels, or infusion of cytotoxic agents such as doxorubicin, cisplatin, or mitomycin C followed by embolization. Embolization can be achieved by gelatin foam, blood clots, or coils. Most clinicians agree that chemo-embolization is more rational than embolization alone despite the lack of randomized trials. The complete necrosis rate of HCCs less than 4 cm treated by TACE is 64%.[123] TACE has a survival advantage over no therapy: 1-year survival, 82% versus 63%; 2-year survival, 63% versus 27%.[124] However, a recent Cochrane database review concluded that there is no current firm evidence to support or refute TACE or bland embolization for patients with unresectable HCC.[125]

   The initial experience for chemoembolization used poppy seed oil, lipidol, as a vehicle to carry the chemotherapeutic agents into the tumor cells. HCC cells are avid for lipidol. The lipidol-cytotoxic emulsion is retained within the tumor cells for weeks. Such retention results in bright white staining on CT images of the infused area, which helps in monitoring the tumor response. Repeat TACE should be based on the tumor response as assessed by CT scans.[126]

   More recently, drug-eluting beads (DEB) have been developed. These are emboliz-ing microparticles that are capable of taking up several drugs such as doxorubicin in vitro by ion exchange and unloading them in vivo.[127] The Barcelona Liver Clinic re-ported improved survival using doxorubicin DEB in Child-Pugh class A and BCLC class A and B.[128]

   The main contraindications for TACE therapy are substantial arteriovenous shunting, main portal vein thrombosis, Child C cirrhosis, and extrahepatic liver metastases. Also, patients with chronic kidney disease cannot tolerate the contrast agent used during the procedure. Some patients experience a self-limiting postembolization syndrome including fever, nausea, and abdominal pain. The complication rate is 23% including liver abscess, tumor rupture, cholecystitis, pancreatitis, peptic ulcer, and renal failure.[129]

Radiation Therapy

Historically, conventional external beam radiotherapy (RT) has not been used for the treatment of HCC because it is not well tolerated by the liver. Damage to the nontumor-bearing liver parenchyma leads to radiation-induced liver disease. It is a syndrome of anicteric hepatomegaly, ascites, and increased transaminases. It can happen 2 weeks and up to 4 months after treatment and may progress to liver failure. The assailant pathologic feature is small vein occlusion with central lobular venous congestion.[130] This led researchers to look for other methods to deliver more focused radiation to the tumor mass.

Transarterial radiotherapy

Traditionally, radioactive iodine (^{131}I) with lipidol has been used to deliver localized radiotherapy to the tumor using a transarterial approach. Complete tumor necrosis was reported in HCC less than 5 cm with superselective high-dose therapy.[131]

In the past decade, radioactive yttrium 90 mounted on microglass beads, microspheres, has been added to the armamentarium of HCC therapy. The ^{90}Y-laden microspheres are delivered via percutaneous hepatic artery catheters directly into the feeding vessels of the tumor. In a European multicenter analysis involving 325 patients with HCC, ^{90}Y therapy showed a survival benefit. Multivariate analysis revealed the most important prognostic factors are the disease stage, Eastern Cooperative Oncology group (ECOG) performance status, INR greater than 1.2, tumor burden (>5 nodules), and extrahepatic disease.[132]

Diffuse intrahepatic HCC is 1 of the major indications for transarterial radiotherapy provided that liver functions are well preserved. Common side effects include fatigue, nausea, vomiting, abdominal pain, cholecystitis, and even liver failure. More serious side effects may result from possible shunting to the lung or the gastrointestinal tract. A pretreatment angiogram and technietium 99m–labeled macroaggregate albumin particles are essential for appropriate patient selection and treatment planning.[133]

Three-dimensional conformal radiotherapy

Three-dimensional conformal radiotherapy (3DCRT) delineates tumors and adjacent normal tissue in 3 dimensions using CT and/or MRI scanners and specialized software. This allows high tumoricidal doses of radiation to be delivered to the tumor with sparing of the surrounding liver parenchyma. Treatment of frail patients with advanced cirrhosis, tumors inaccessible to percutaneous ablative modalities (eg, close to the diaphragm), and patients with portal vein tumor thrombosis (PVTT) is possible. In a phase 2 study, 3DCRT was applied in a dose of 66 Gy, 2 Gy daily to tumors 2 cm to 6.5 cm; the objective response rate was 80% to 92%.[134] Reactivation of HBV has been reported following 3DCRT for HCC.[135] Another interesting phenomenon is that most recurrences after focal radiotherapy are outside the radiated field as a result of rapid progression of the dormant subclinical tumors. One of the proposed underlying mechanisms is upregulation of vascular endothelial growth factor (VEGF) secondary to radiation injury of the vascular endothelium.[136]

The next generation of 3DCRT is intensity-modulated radiotherapy, which is an advanced high-precision radiation. It improves the ability to conform the radiotherapy to the tumor shape.[137]

Another strategy to deliver radiotherapy is stereotactic body radiation therapy (SBRT). Tse and colleagues[138] treated 31 patients with a median tumor volume of 73 mL with a median dose of 36 Gy in 6 fractions of SBRT. The median survival was 11.7 months.

Proton beam radiotherapy

In proton beam radiotherapy (PBR), protons passing near the electrons orbiting the nuclei of cancer cells pull the electrons out of their orbits, interfering with their ability to proliferate. It can be applied in 3D patterns with great precision. The dose is reported in cobalt Gray equivalents (GyE). Preliminary results of this emerging technology are promising despite the cost and scarcity of PBR machines. In 1 series of 79 patients with HCC, the median dose was 72 GyE in 16 fractions. At 5 years, the rate of local control was 89% and survival was 27%.[139] Eradication of HCC by PBR was shown in explanted livers. In a series of 18 patients who underwent liver transplant after having received PBR 2 to 55 months before transplant at a dose of 63 GyE in 15 fractions over 3 weeks, 6 (33%) patients showed complete pathologic response.[140]

Combined Locoregional Therapies

In the quest for complete tumor necrosis, TACE has been combined with local ablative therapies.

Combining TACE with PEI helps to slow down the washout effect of circulating blood on the locally injected ethanol, hence increasing ethanol diffusion and the tumoricidal effect. In 1 study that compared TACE alone with combined TACE and PEI, the latter showed a significantly higher complete response rate and a superior recurrence-free survival.[141]

The rational of combining TACE with thermal ablative therapies is that embolization of tumor feeding vessels eliminates the cooling effect of circulating blood in the tumor making thermal therapies more effective. Interruption of the tumor blood supply followed by RFA achieved a 90% response rate.[142]

3DCRT was combined with TACE in patients with PVTT. In a series of 412 patients treated with TACE followed by a median radiation dose of 40 Gy delivered in 2- to 5-Gy fractions, the objective PVTT response rate was 39.6% and the tumor-free progression rate was 85.6%. Patients' median survival was 10.6 months. Hepatic toxicity and gastroduodenal complications were observed in 10% and 3.6% of patients, respectively.[143]

Systemic Chemotherapy

Systemic chemotherapy with cytotoxic agents has been disappointing in the treatment of HCC, yielding a response rate of 10% to 20% but no overall survival benefit. Doxorubicin is the most commonly used agent in systemic therapy for HCC. In a phase 3 trial comparing doxorubicin with nolatrexed, the objective response rate of doxorubicin was 4% versus 1.4%.[144]

An aggressive combination regimen, PIAF (cisplatin, interferon alfa-2b, doxorubicin, and 5-fluoruracil) has shown a response rate of 26% and a median survival of approximately 9 months in a single-arm phase 2 trial.[145] Despite confirming the response rate of the PIAF regimen in a randomized phase 3 study comparing doxorubicin alone versus PIAF with a reported response rate of 10.5% versus 20.9%, the median survival difference was not significant: 6.8 months versus 8.6 months, respectively.[146] However, multiple experts panels concluded that underlying liver disease is a major confounding factor that independently affects HCC treatment outcome. This fact is pertinent to failed chemotherapy trials in HCC because most patients did not tolerate full doses and regular schedules of chemotherapy, and therefore, the poor outcome and short survival time were related, in part, to deterioration of the underlying liver disease. Notably, Kaseb and colleagues[147] most recently reported a 36% response rate and 33% rate of conversion to curative surgery in a cohort of 33 patients with HCC and no significant cirrhosis. However, prospective randomized trials in patients with HCC and no significant cirrhosis is warranted to confirm the usefulness of the PIAF regimen as a potential neoadjuvant therapy.

Molecular Targeted Therapies

Hepatocarcinogenesis engages compound, diverse, signaling pathways. Targeting molecules with agents that have multiple signaling pathway effects has become an interesting field in HCC therapy.

Sorafenib is an oral multikinase inhibitor that blocks tumor cell proliferation by targeting raf/MEK/ERK signaling. It also has antiangiogenic properties by targeting VEGF receptor-2/-3 and platelet-derived growth factor (PDGF) β-tyrosine kinases.[148] Sorafenib has been approved as the standard of care for advanced unresectable HCC. It should be used cautiously because of its side effects, primarily hand and feet skin exfoliation, fatigue, and hepatic toxicity. A phase 3 clinical trial, the Sorafenib HCC Assessment Randomized Protocol (SHARP) study, including 602 patients with advanced HCC, compared sorafineb with placebo. Child-Pugh class A cirrhosis was prevalent in 95% of the sorafineb group and 98% of the placebo group. Sorafineb showed significant benefit in terms of median overall survival in the sorafineb arm of 10.6 months versus 7.9 months for the placebo arm ($P<.001$) and a 31% decrease in the death rate in the sorafineb arm.[149]

Select inhibitors of the angiogenic pathway

The VEGF and PDGF families are involved in angiogenesis, a key in the development of HCC.

Bevacizumab, a recombinant humanized monoclonal antibody that targets VEGF, has become an effective therapy in many cancers. Twenty-five patients were evaluated in a phase 1 trial using bevacizumab as a single agent for the treatment of inoperable HCC without metastases or macrovascular invasion. Two patients had partial response and 18 patients had stable disease.[150] Subsequently, the signal of activity of bevacizumab in HCC was reported in phase 2 studies, either alone or combined with erlotinib.[151–154]

In addition, in a phase 2 trial, bevacizumab was used in combination with capecitabine and oxaliplatin in patients with advanced HCC. Eleven percent of patients evaluated had partial response and 78% had sustained response.[155] Side effects of bevacizumab include bleeding, hypertension, and proteinuria.

FUTURE THERAPIES UNDER INVESTIGATION

Solid tumors develop after disruption of at least 3 critical intracellular signaling pathways.[156–158] Encouraged by the success of sorafineb in the treatment of inoperable HCCs and motivated by a subgroup of patients who are refractory to sorafineb, other molecular targeted therapies are under development in clinical trials.

Select Approaches of Molecular Targeted Therapies

c-MET inhibitors

A recent example of the personalized targeted therapy approach in HCC is represented by data from a study of tivantinib (ARQ 197), an oral inhibitor of MET. Tivantinib was found to have promising activity in HCC as monotherapy in a randomized, placebo-controlled, double-blind, phase 2 study as a second-line treatment of advanced HCC. Forty-six (65%) patients in the tivantinib group and 26 (72%) of those in the placebo group had progressive disease. Time to progression was longer for patients treated with tivantinib (1.6 months [95% CI 1.4–2.8]) than placebo (1.4 months [1.4–1.5]; hazard ratio [HR] 0.64, 90% CI 0.43–0.94; $P = .04$). For patients with MET-high tumors by immunohistochemistry, median time to progression was longer in patients treated with tivantinib than for those treated with placebo (2.7 months

[95% CI 1.4–8.5] for 22 tivantinib patients vs 1.4 months [1.4–1.6] for 15 placebo patients; HR 0.43, 95% CI 0.19–0.97; P = .03). A phase 3 trial is underway to confirm the activity of tivantinib in c-MET high patients.[159]

Epidermal growth factor receptor inhibitors

Epidermal growth factor receptor (EGFR) was found in 16 of 25 (64%) less-differentiated HCCs and 17 of 24 (71%) adjacent nontumor liver parenchyma.[160] Several EGFR tyrosine kinase inhibitors have been investigated in HCC therapy.

Erlotinib was studied in a phase 2 trial including 38 patients with advanced HCC. After 6 months of therapy, 32 patients were progression free, with a median progression-free survival of 3.8 months. The most frequent side effects were skin rash, diarrhea, and fatigue. Nevertheless, immunohistochemical staining for EGFR expression did not have an effect on the outcome.[161]

Lapatinib a dual inhibitor of EGFR tyrosine kinase 1and 2 has been studied in a phase 2 trial enrolling 30 patients with advanced HCC. The median progression-free survival was 1.8 months.[162]

Cetuximab, a chimeric monoclonal antibody against EGFR, was investigated in 2 phase 2 studies. In 1 cohort of 30 patients, the median overall survival was 9.6 months (95% CI 4.3–12.1) and the median progression-free survival was 1.4 months (95% CI 1.2–2.6 months).[163] In the other study, 27 patients were evaluated but no response was observed.[164]

These data are limited by the small number of patients in small single-institution phase 2 studies.

Irreversible Electroporation (NanoKnife)

Irreversible electroporation (IRE) is a developing technology for tumor ablation. It creates a nanoscale cell membrane defect through the delivery of intense electrical pulses up to 3000 V. It has been validated in an animal model.[165] The advantage of this innovative technology is that it does not produce intense heat and therefore can be applied to tumors adjacent to bile ducts and blood vessels. Also, the ablated area has well-defined boundaries compared with surrounding nonablated tissue. The safety of IRE has been examined in 38 patients with a total of 69 advanced liver, kidney, and lung tumors. One of the major side effects was transient ventricular arrhythmia in 4 patients, which was overcome by electrocardiographic synchronized delivery. Total tumor response, assessed by CT scan, was achieved in 66% of the tumors with a better response in liver tumors.[166]

Gene Therapy

In the past decade, gene therapy approaches to HCC have been under experimental investigation. Gene therapy is a diverse field that encompasses a wide variety of therapeutic genes, vectors both viral and nonviral, routes of administration, and regulatory sequences all of which can be used alone or in combination. The progress of gene therapy has been tampered by researchers' caution and spectators' skepticism because of possible serious side effects. Gene therapy in HCC involves intracellular transfer of genetic material such as apoptotic genes mediating cell death, oncolytic viral vectors, genes coding for inhibition of angiogenesis, genetic prodrug activation, genetic immunotherapy, and small interfering RNA (siRNA) targeted gene silencing.[167,168] Encouraging results in ex vivo and animal models have been difficult to translate to patients because such models cannot reiterate the key features in human hepatocarcinogenesis. Evolving clinical trials are in phase 1 and 2. Details of such trials are beyond the scope of this article and can be reviewed at www.genetherapynet.com.

Circulating Tumor Cells

Recurrence is 1 of the major challenges after curative cancer therapy. The concept of circulating tumor cells (CTCs) is strongly suggested by more than 10% recurrence of HCC, mostly in the allograft, after liver transplant.[101] Detection of CTCs can be achieved by (1) tumor-specific nucleic acid analysis such as using reverse transcriptase polymerase chain reaction liver-specific human AFP mRNA, (2) cytometric analysis using immunohistochemistry to detect antibodies against various epithelial-specific antigens and flow cytometry, and (3) functional analysis by detection of specific marker proteins secreted by the tumor cells.[169] In a series of 85 patients with HCC, CTCs were detected in 81% of patients and highly correlated with tumor-node metastases (TNM) staging.[170] This concept is open to a wide range of clinical implications such as staging, treatment strategies, and patient selection for liver transplant.

SUMMARY

Management of HCC is a rapidly evolving field. In the past decade, with advances in liver surgery and transplantation, curative treatment can be offered to patients with HCC in compensated livers who are diagnosed early or to those who are within transplant criteria. Explanted livers have provided a growing understanding of the underlying mechanisms in hepatocarcinogenesis and diagnostic modalities. For those tumors not amenable to resection or transplantation, several locoregional therapies are available. For advanced tumors, molecular targeted therapies are yielding promising results. Because of the heterogeneity of the patients and the disease, many questions are waiting for answers through well-designed, adequately powered, and bias-free multicenter, controlled, randomized trials.

REFERENCES

1. Centre for Disease Control and Prevention (CDC). Hepatocellular carcinoma in the United States, 2001–2006. MMWR Morb Mortal Wkly Rep 2010;59(17):517–20.
2. El-Serag HB, Rudolph KL. Hepatocellular carcinoma: epidemiology and molecular carcinogenesis. Gastroenterology 2007;132:2557–76.
3. Carreno V, Bartolome J, Castillo I, et al. Occult hepatitis B virus and hepatitis C virus infections. Rev Med Virol 2008;18:139–57.
4. Abdel-Aziz F, Habib M, Mohamed MK, et al. Hepatitis C virus (HCV) infection in a community in the Nile Delta: population description and HCV prevalence. Hepatology 2000;32:111–5.
5. Kim CM, Koike K, Saito I, et al. HBX gene of hepatitis B virus induced liver cancer in transgenic mice. Nature 1991;351:317–20.
6. Truant R, Antunovic J, Greenblatt J, et al. Direct interaction of hepatitis B virus HBX protein with p53 leads to inhibition by HBx of p 53 response element-directed transactivation. J Virol 1995;69:1851–9.
7. Chang M, Chen C, Mei-Shu Lai M, et al. Universal hepatitis B vaccination in Taiwan and the incidence of hepatocellular carcinoma in children. Taiwan Childhood Hepatoma Study Group. N Engl J Med 1997;336:1855–9.
8. Cammà C, Giunta M, Andreone P, et al. Interferon and prevention of hepatocellular carcinoma in viral cirrhosis: an evidence-based approach. J Hepatol 2001; 34(4):593–602.
9. International Agency for Research on Cancer. Hepatitis viruses. In: IARC monographs on the evaluation of carcinogenic risks to humans, vol. 59. Lyon (France): IARC; 1994.

10. Verme G, Brunetto MR, Oliveri F, et al. Role of hepatitis delta virus infection in hepatocellular carcinoma. Dig Dis Sci 1991;36:1134–6.
11. Degos F, Christidis C, Ganne-Carrie N, et al. Hepatitis C virus related cirrhosis: time to occurrence of hepatocellular carcinoma and death. Gut 2000;47:131–6.
12. Kew MC. Hepatitis B and C viruses and hepatocellular carcinoma. Clin Lab Med 1996;16:395–406.
13. Friedman S. Mechanisms of disease: mechanisms of hepatic fibrosis and therapeutic implications. Nat Clin Pract Gastroenterol Hepatol 2004;1:98–105.
14. Koshy R, Maupas P, Muller R, et al. Detection of hepatitis B virus-specific DNA in the genomes of human hepatocellular carcinoma and liver cirrhosis tissues. J Gen Virol 1981;57(Pt 1):95–102.
15. Xu Z, Jensen G, Yen TS. Activation of hepatitis B virus S promoter by the viral large surface protein via induction of stress in the endoplasmic reticulum. J Virol 1997;71:7387–92.
16. Donato F, Tagger A, Gelatti U, et al. Alcohol and hepatocellular carcinoma: the effect of lifetime intake and hepatitis virus infections in men and women. Am J Epidemiol 2002;155:323–31.
17. Morgan TR, Mandayam S, Jamal MM. Alcohol and hepatocellular carcinoma. Gastroenterology 2004;127(5 Suppl 1):S87–96.
18. Callee EE, Rodriguez C, Walker-Thurmond K, et al. Overweight, obesity and mortality from cancer in a prospective studied cohort of US adults. N Engl J Med 2003;348:1625–38.
19. Hassan M, Hwang L, Hatten CJ, et al. Risk factors for hepatocellular carcinoma: synergism of alcohol with viral hepatitis and diabetes mellitus. Hepatology 2002; 36(5):1206–13.
20. Shimada M, Hashimoto E, Taniai M, et al. Hepatocellular carcinoma in patients with non-alcoholic steatohepatitis. J Hepatol 2002;37:154–60.
21. McCollough AJ. The clinical features, diagnosis and natural history of non-alcoholic fatty liver disease. Clin Liver Dis 2004;8:521–33.
22. Finch SC, Finch CA. Idiopathic hemochromatosis and iron storage disease: A. Iron metabolism in hemochromatosis. Medicine 1995;34:381–430.
23. Bassendine M, Rushbrook S, Chapman R, et al, editors. Primary Biliary Cirrhosis. Sherlock's diseases of the liver and biliary system. 12th edition. Edinburgh (United Kingdom): Blackwell Science; 2011. p. 338–42.
24. Farinati F, Floreani A, De Maria N, et al. Hepatocellular carcinoma in primary biliary cirrhosis. J Hepatol 1994;21(3):315–6.
25. Hassan MM, Zaghloul AS, El-Serag HB, et al. The role of hepatitis C in hepatocellular carcinoma: a case control study among Egyptian patients. J Clin Gastroenterol 2001;33:123–6.
26. Takayasu K, Muramatsu Y, Moriyama N, et al. Radiological study of idiopathic Budd-Chiari syndrome complicated by hepatocellular carcinoma. A report of four cases. Am J Gastroenterol 1994;89(2):249–53.
27. Havlioglu N, Brunt EM, Bacon BR. Budd-Chiari syndrome and hepatocellular carcinoma: a case report and review of the literature. Am J Gastroenterol 2003;98:201–4.
28. Belghiti J, Vilgrain V, Paradis V. Benign liver lesions. In: Blumgart LH, editor. Surgery of the liver and biliary tract and the pancreas. 4th edition. Edniburgh (United Kingdom): Saunders; 2007. p. 1142–3.
29. Bioulac-Sage P, Laumonier H, Couchy G, et al. Hepatology 2009;50(2):481–9.
30. Bioulac-Sage P, Rebouissou S, Thomas C, et al. Hepatology 2007;46(3):740–8.

31. Liu Y, Chang CC, Marsh GM, et al. Population attributable risk of aflatoxin-related liver cancer: systematic review and meta-analysis. Eur J Cancer 2012; 48(14):2125–36.
32. Kuper H, Tzonou A, Kaklamani E, et al. Tobacco smoking, alcohol consumption and their interaction in the causation of hepatocellular carcinoma. Int J Cancer 2000;85(4):498–502.
33. Trevisani F, Cantarini MC, Labate AM, et al. Surveillance for hepatocellular carcinoma in elderly Italian patients with cirrhosis: effects on cancer staging and patient survival. Am J Gastroenterol 2004;99:1470–6.
34. Wong V, Chan S, Mo F, et al. Clinical scoring system to predict hepatocellular carcinoma in chronic hepatitis B carriers. J Clin Oncol 2010;28(10):1660–5.
35. Imbert-Bismut F, Ratziu V, Pieroni L, et al. Biochemical markers of liver fibrosis in patients with hepatitis C virus infection: a prospective study. Lancet 2001;357: 1069–75.
36. Moriyama M, Matsumura H, Aoki H, et al. Long-term outcome, with monitoring of platelet counts, in patients with chronic hepatitis C and liver cirrhosis after interferon therapy. Intervirology 2003;46:296–307.
37. Befrits R, Hedman M, Blomquist L, et al. Chronic hepatitis C in alcoholic patients: prevalence, genotypes, and correlation to liver disease. Scand J Gastroenterol 1995;30:1113–8.
38. Ong JP, Pitts A, Younossi ZM. Increased overall mortality and liver-related mortality in non-alcoholic fatty liver disease. J Hepatol 2008;49:608–12.
39. Silveira MG, Suzuki A, Lindor KD. Surveillance for hepatocellular carcinoma in patients with primary biliary cirrhosis. Hepatology 2008;48(4):1149–56.
40. Fracanzani AL, Conte D, Fraquelli M, et al. Increased cancer risk in a cohort of 230 patients with hereditary hemochromatosis in comparison to matched control patients with non-iron related chronic liver disease. Hepatology 2001;33:647–51.
41. Izzo F, Cremona F, Ruffolo F, et al. Outcome of 67 patients with hepatocellular cancer detected during screening of 1125 patients with chronic hepatitis. Ann Surg 1998;227:513–8.
42. Sherman M. Surveillance for hepatocellular carcinoma and early diagnosis. Clin Liver Dis 2007;11:817–37.
43. Peterson M, Baron R, Marsh W Jr, et al. Pretransplantation surveillance for possible hepatocellular carcinoma in patients with cirrhosis: epidemiology and CT-based tumor detection rate in 430 cases with surgical pathologic correlation. Radiology 2000;217:743–9.
44. Bolondi L, Sofia S, Siringo S, Gaiani S, et al. Surveillance programme of cirrhotic patients for early diagnosis and treatment of hepatocellular carcinoma: a cost-effectiveness analysis. Gut 2001;48:251–9.
45. Masuzaki R, Tateishi R, Yoshida H, et al. Prospective risk assessment for hepatocellular carcinoma development in patients with chronic hepatitis C by transient elastography. Hepatology 2009;49(6):296–307.
46. Burix J, Sherman M. Management of hepatocellular carcinoma. AASLD practice guidelines. Hepatology 2005;42(5):1208–36.
47. Burix J, Sherman M. Management of hepatocellular carcinoma: an update. Hepatology 2011;53(3):1020–2.
48. Sato Y, Sekine T, Ohwada S. Alpha-fetoprotein-producing rectal cancer: calculated tumor marker doubling time. J Surg Oncol 1994;55:265–8.
49. Adachi Y, Tsuchihashi J, Shiraishi N, et al. AFP-producing gastric carcinoma: multivariate analysis of prognostic factors in 270 patients. Oncology 2003;65: 95–101.

50. Li D, Mallorya T, Satomurab S. AFP-L3: a new generation of tumor marker for hepatocellular carcinoma. Clin Chim Acta 2001;313(1–2):15–9.
51. Paradis V, Degos F, Dargere D, et al. Identification of a new marker of hepatocellular carcinoma by serum protein profiling of patients with chronic liver diseases. Hepatology 2005;41:40–7.
52. Lok A, Sterling R, Everhart J, et al. HALT-C Trial Group. Des-γ-carboxy prothrombin and α-fetoprotein as biomarkers for the early detection of hepatocellular carcinoma. Gastroenterology 2010;138(2):493–502.
53. Zinkin N, Grall F, Bhaskar K, et al. Serum proteomics and biomarkers in hepatocellular carcinoma and chronic liver disease. Clin Cancer Res 2008;15(14):470.
54. Bennett GL, Krinsky G, Abitbol R, et al. Sonographic detection of hepatocellular carcinoma and dysplastic nodules in cirrhosis. Correlation of pretransplantation sonography and liver explant pathology in 200 patients. AJR Am J Roentgenol 2002;179:75–80.
55. Wilson SR, Burns PN, Muradali D, et al. Harmonic hepatic US with microbubble contrast agent: initial experience showing improved characterization of hemangioma, hepatocellular carcinoma, and metastasis. Radiology 2000;215:153–61.
56. Kim T, Murakami T, Takahashi S, et al. Optimal phases of dynamic CT for detecting hepatocellular carcinoma: evaluation of unenhanced and triple-phase images. Abdom Imaging 1999;24:473–80.
57. Ito K. Hepatocellular carcinoma: conventional MRI findings including gadolinium-enhanced dynamic imaging. Eur J Radiol 2006;58(2):186–99.
58. Yamshita Y, Mitsuzaki K, Yi T, et al. Small hepatocellular carcinoma in patient with chronic liver damage: prospective comparison of detection with dynamic MR imaging and helical CT of the whole liver. Radiology 1996;200:79–84.
59. Shimizu A, Ito K, Koike S, et al. Cirrhosis or chronic hepatitis: evaluation of small (or 2-cm) early-enhancing hepatic lesions with serial contrast-enhanced dynamic MR imaging. Radiology 2003;226:550–5.
60. Kashiwagi T. PDG-PET and hepatocellular carcinoma. J Gastroenterol 2004;39: 1017–8.
61. Stigliano R, Marelli L, Yu D, et al. Seeding following percutaneous diagnostic and therapeutic approaches for hepatocellular carcinoma. What is the risk and the outcome? Seeding risk for percutaneous approach of HCC. Cancer Treat Rev 2007;33(5):437–47.
62. Child CG, Turcotte JG. Surgery and portal hypertension. In: Child CG, editor. The liver and portal hypertension. Philadelphia: Saunders; 1964. p. 50–64.
63. Pugh RN, Murray-Lyon IM, Dawson JL, et al. Transection of the oesophagus for bleeding oesophageal varices. Br J Surg 1973;60:648–52.
64. Okuda K, Ohtsuki T, Obata H, et al. Natural history of hepatocellular carcinoma and prognosis in relation to treatment. Study of 850 patients. Cancer 1985;56: 918–28.
65. Malinchoc M, Kamath P, Gordon F, et al. A model to predict poor survival in patients undergoing transjugular portosystemic shunts. Hepatology 2000;31:864–71.
66. Llovet JM, Bru C, Bruix J. Prognosis of hepatocellular carcinoma: the BCLC staging classification. Semin Liver Dis 1999;19:329–38.
67. Wildi S, Petalozzi B, McCormack L, et al. Critical evaluation of the different staging systems for hepatocellular carcinoma. Br J Surg 2004;91:400–8.
68. Llovet JM, Burroughs A, Bruix J. Hepatocellular carcinoma. Lancet 2003; 362(9399):1907–17.
69. Llovet JM. Updated treatment approach to hepatocellular carcinoma. J Gastroenterol 2005;40:225–35.

70. Llovet JX, Bruix J, Gores GJ. Surgical resection versus transplantation for early he-patocellular carcinoma. Clues for the best therapy. Hepatology 2000;31:1019–21.
71. Yamanaka J, Saito S, Fujimoto J. Impact of preoperative planning using virtual segmental volumetry on liver resection for hepatocellular carcinoma. World J Surg 2007;31:1249–55.
72. Vauthey JN, Chaoui A, Do KA. Standardized measurement of the future liver remnant prior to extended liver resection: methodology and clinical association. Surgery 2000;127:512–9.
73. Hashimoto M, Watanabe G. Hepatic parenchymal cell volume and the indocya-nine green tolerance test. J Surg Res 2000;92:222–7.
74. Fong Y, Sun RL, Jarnagin W, et al. An analysis of 412 cases of hepatocellular carcinoma at a Western center. Ann Surg 1999;229:790–9.
75. Imamura H, Matsuyama Y, Tanaka E, et al. Risk factors contributing to early and late phase intrahepatic recurrence of hepatocellular carcinoma after hepatec-tomy. J Hepatol 2003;38:200–7.
76. Maithel SK, Kneuertz PJ, Kooby DA, et al. Importance of low preoperative platelet count in selecting patients for resection of hepatocellular carcinoma: a multi-institutional analysis. J Am Coll Surg 2011;212(4):638–48 [discussion: 648–50].
77. Makuuchi M, Thai BL, Takayasu K, et al. Preoperative portal embolization to in-crease safety of major hepatectomy for hilar bile duct carcinoma: a preliminary report. Surgery 1990;107:521–7.
78. Kokudo N, Makuuchi M. Current role of portal vein embolization/hepatic artery chemoembolization. Surg Clin North Am 2004;84:643–57.
79. Abdalla EK, Hicks ME, Vauthey JN. Portal vein embolization: rationale, tech-nique and future prospects. Br J Surg 2001;88:165–75.
80. Ribero D, Abdalla E, Madoff D, et al. Portal vein embolization before major hep-atectomy and its effects on regeneration, resectability and outcome. Br J Surg 2007;94:1386–94.
81. Nagino M, Nimura Y, Kamiya J, et al. Immediate increase in arterial blood flow in embolized hepatic segments after portal vein embolization: CT demonstration. Am J Roentgenol 1998;171:1037–9.
82. Aoki K, Imamura H, Hasegawa K, et al. Sequential Preoperative arterial and por-tal venous embolizations in patients with hepatocellular carcinoma. Arch Surg 2004;139:766–74.
83. Abulkhir A, Limongelli P, Healey AJ, et al. Preoperative portal vein embolization for major liver resection: a meta-analysis. Ann Surg 2008;247(1):49–57.
84. Pai M, Zacharoulis D, Milicevic MN, et al. Autologous infusion of expanded mobilized adult bone marrow-derived CD34+ cells into patients with alcoholic liver cirrhosis. Am J Gastroenterol 2008;103(8):1952–8.
85. am Esch JS 2nd, Knoefel WT, Klein M, et al. Portal application of autologous CD133+ bone marrow cells to the liver: a novel concept to support hepatic regeneration. Stem Cells 2005;23(4):463–70.
86. Stremitzer S, Tamandl D, Kaczirek K, et al. Value of hepatic venous pressure gradient measurement before liver resection for hepatocellular carcinoma. Br J Surg 2011;98(12):1752–8.
87. Boleslawski E, Petrovai G, Truant S, et al. Hepatic venous pressure gradient in the assessment of portal hypertension before liver resection in patients with cirrhosis. Br J Surg 2012;99(6):855–63.
88. Cherqui D, Laurent A, Tayar C, et al. Laparoscopic liver resection for peripheral hepatocellular carcinoma in patients with chronic liver disease midterm results and perspectives. Ann Surg 2006;243(4):499–502.

89. Jiao LR, Ayav A, Navarra G, et al. Laparoscopic liver resection assisted by the laparoscopic Habib Sealer. Surgery 2008;144(5):770–4.

90. Azoulay D, Andreani P, Maggi U. Combined liver resection and reconstruction of the supra- renal vena cava: the Paul Brousse experience. Ann Surg 2006;244: 80–8.

91. Lang H, Radtke A, Hindennach M, et al. Impact of virtual tumor resection and computer-assisted risk analysis on operation planning and intraoperative strategy in major hepatic resection. Arch Surg 2005;140:629–38.

92. Clinical Trials. Evaluation of image-guided liver surgical system for resection of liver cancer. US National Institute of Health. Available at: http://clinicaltrials.gov/ct2/show/NCT00782886.

93. Mazzaferro V, Regalia E, Doci R, et al. Liver transplantation for the treatment of small hepatocellular carcinomas in patients with cirrhosis. N Engl J Med 1996; 334:693–9.

94. Breitenstein S, Dimitroulis D, Petrowsky H, et al. Systematic review and meta-analysis of interferon after curative treatment of hepatocellular carcinoma in patients with viral hepatitis. Br J Surg 2009;96:975–81.

95. Iwatzuki S, Gordon R, Sahw B Jr, et al. Role of liver transplantation in cancer therapy. Ann Surg 1985;202(40):401–7.

96. Yao FY, Ferrell L, Bass NM, et al. Liver transplantation for hepatocellular carcinoma: expansion of the tumor size limits does not adversely impact survival. Hepatology 2001;33:1394–403.

97. Adler M, De Pauw F, Vereerstraeten P, et al. Outcome of patients with hepatocellular carcinoma listed for liver transplantation within the Eurotransplant allocation system. Liver Transpl 2008;14:526–33.

98. DuBay D, Sandroussi C, Sandhu L, et al. Liver transplantation for advanced hepatocellular carcinoma using poor tumor differentiation on biopsy as an exclusion criterion. Ann Surg 2011;253:166–72.

99. Rougier P, Mitrya E, Barbareb JC, et al. Hepatocellular carcinoma (HCC): an update. Semin Oncol 2007;34(Suppl 1):S12–20.

100. Singhal A, Jayaraman M, Dhanasekaran D, et al. Molecular and serum markers in hepatocellular carcinoma: predictive tools for prognosis and recurrence. Crit Rev Oncol Hematol 2012;82(2):116–40.

101. Mazzaferro V, Llovet JM, Miceli R, et al. Predicting survival after liver transplantation in patients with hepatocellular carcinoma beyond the Milan criteria: a retrospective, exploratory analysis. Lancet Oncol 2009;10:35–43.

102. Yao FY, Hirose R, LaBerge JM. A prospective study on downstaging hepatocellular carcinoma prior to liver transplantation. Liver Transpl 2005;11: 505–14.

103. Graziadei I, Sandmueller H, Waldenberger P, et al. Chemoembolization followed by liver transplantation for hepatocellular carcinoma impedes tumor progression while on the waiting list and leads to excellent outcome. Liver Transpl 2003;9(6): 557–63.

104. United Network of Organ Sharing. Available at: http://www.unos.org.

105. Klintmalm GB, Davis GL, Teperman L, et al. A randomized, multicenter study comparing steroid-free immunosuppression and standard immunosuppression for liver transplant recipients with chronic hepatitis C. Liver Transpl 2011; 17(12):1394–403.

106. Toso C, Merani S, Bigam D, et al. Sirolimus-based immunosuppression is associated with increased survival after liver transplantation for hepatocellular carcinoma. Hepatology 2009;51(4):1237–43.

107. Decaens T, Roudot-Thoraval F, Bresson-Handi S, et al. Role of immunosuppression and tumor differentiation in predicting recurrence after liver transplantation for hepatocellular carcinoma: a multicenter study of 412 patients. World J Gastroenterol 2006;12(45):7319–25.

108. Vakili K, Pomposelli JJ, Cheah YL, et al. Living donor liver transplantation for hepatocellular carcinoma: increased recurrence but improved survival. Liver Transpl 2009;15:1861–6.

109. Montorsi M, Santambrogio R, Bianchi P, et al. Radiofrequency interstitial thermal ablation of hepatocellular carcinoma in liver cirrhosis. Role of the laparoscopic approach. Surg Endosc 2001;15:141–5.

110. Curley S, Izzo F, Ellis LM, et al. Radiofrequency ablation of hepatocellular carcinoma in 110 patients with cirrhosis. Ann Surg 2000;232:381–91.

111. Siperstein AE, Rogers SJ, Hansen PD, et al. Laparoscopic thermal ablation of hepatic neuroendocrine tumor metastases. Surgery 1997;122:1147–55.

112. Wood TF, Rose DM, Chung M, et al. Radiofrequency ablation of 231 unresectable hepatic tumours: indications, limitations and complications. Ann Surg Oncol 2000;7:593–600.

113. Solbiati L, Goldberg SN, Ierace T, et al. Radio-frequency ablation of hepatic metastases: postprocedural assessment with a US microbubble contrast agent— early experience. Radiology 1999;211:643–9.

114. Khorsandi S, Kysela P, Valek V, et al. Initial data on a novel endovascular radiofrequency catheter when used for arterial occlusion in liver cancer. Eur Surg 2009;41(3):104–8.

115. Shina S, Tagawa K, Unuma T, et al. Percutaneous ethanol injection therapy for hepatocellular carcinoma. A histopathologic study. Cancer 1991;68: 1524–30.

116. Livraghi T, Golberg SN, Lazzaroni S, et al. Small hepatocellular carcinoma: treatment with radiofrequency ablation versus percutaneous ethanol injection. Radiology 1999;210:655–61.

117. Hyodoh H, Hyodoh K, Takahashi K, et al. Microwave coagulation therapy on hepatomas: CT and MR appearance after therapy. J Magn Reson Imaging 1998;2:451–8.

118. Seki S, Sakaguchi H, Kadoya H, et al. Laparoscopic microwave coagulation therapy for hepatocellular carcinoma. Endoscopy 2000;32:591–7.

119. Giorgio A, Tarantino L, de Stefano G, et al. Interstitial laser photocoagulation under ultrasound guidance of liver tumors: results in 104treated patients. Eur J Ultrasound 2000;11:181–8.

120. Wren SM, Coburn MM, Tan M, et al. Is cryosurgical ablation appropriate for treating hepatocellular cancer? Arch Surg 1997;132:599–603.

121. Seifert JK, Morris DL. World survey on the complications of hepatic and prostate cryotherapy. World J Surg 1999;23:109–14.

122. Majno PE, Adam R, Bismuth H, et al. Influence of preoperative transarterial Lipiodol chemoembolization on resection and transplantation for hepatocellular carcinoma in patients with cirrhosis. Ann Surg 1997;226:688–703.

123. Matsui O, Kadoya M, Yoshikawa J, et al. Subsegmental transcatheter arterial embolization for small hepatocellular carcinomas: local therapeutic effect and 5-year survival rate. Cancer Chemother Pharmacol 1994;33(Suppl):S84–8.

124. Llovet JM, Real MI, Montaña X, et al, Barcelona Liver Cancer Group. Arterial embolisation or chemo-embolisation versus symptomatic treatment in patients with unresectable hepatocellular carcinoma: a randomised controlled trial. Lancet 2002;359(9319):1734–9.

125. Oliveri RS, Wetterslev J, Gluud C. Transarterial (chemo)embolisation for unresectable hepatocellular carcinoma. Cochrane Database Syst Rev 2011;(3):CD004787.

126. Ernst O, Sergent G, Mizrahi D, et al. Treatment of hepatocellular carcinoma by transcatheter arterial chemoembolization: comparison of planned periodic chemoembolization and chemoembolization based on tumor response. Am J Roentgenol 1999;172:59–64.

127. Varela M, Real MI, Burrel M, et al. Chemoembolization of hepatocellular carcinoma with drug eluting beads: efficacy and doxorubicin pharmacokinetics. J Hepatol 2007;46:474–81.

128. Burrel M, Reig M, Forner A, et al. Survival of patients with hepatocellular carcinoma treated by transarterial chemoembolisation (TACE) using drug eluting beads. Implications for clinical practice and trial design. J Hepatol 2012; 56(6):1330–5.

129. Poon RT, Ngan H, Lo CM, et al. Transarterial chemoembolization for inoperable hepatocellular carcinoma and postresection intrahepatic recurrence. J Surg Oncol 2000;73:109–14.

130. Yoo HS, Park CH, Lee JT, et al. Small hepatocellular carcinoma: high dose internal radiation therapy with superselective intra-arterial injection of I-131-labeled Lipiodol. Cancer Chemother Pharmacol 1994;33(Suppl):S128–33.

131. Sangro B, Carpanese L, Cianni R, et al, European Network on Radioembolization with Yttrium-90 Resin Microspheres (ENRY). Survival after yttrium-90 resin microsphere radioembolization of hepatocellular carcinoma across Barcelona clinic liver cancer stages: a European evaluation. Hepatology 2011;54(3): 868–78.

132. Kennedy A, Coldwell D, Sangro B, et al. Radioembolization for the treatment of liver tumors general principles. Am J Clin Oncol 2012;35(1):91–9.

133. Dawson LA, Normolle D, Balter JM, et al. Analysis of radiation-induced liver disease using the Lyman NTCP model. Int J Radiat Oncol Biol Phys 2002;53(4): 810–21.

134. Mornex F, Girard N, Beziat C, et al. Feasibility and efficacy of high-dose three-dimensional conformal radiotherapy in cirrhotic patients with small-size hepatocellular carcinoma noneligible for curative therapies –mature results of the French phase-II RTF-1 trial. Int J Radiat Oncol Biol Phys 2006;66:1152–8.

135. Kim JH, Park JW, Kim TH, et al. Hepatitis B virus reactivation after three-dimensional conformal radiotherapy in patients with hepatitis B virus related hepatocellular carcinoma. Int J Radiat Oncol Biol Phys 2007;69(3):813–9.

136. Chung YL, Jian JJ, Cheng SH, et al. Sublethal irradiation induces vascular endothelial growth factor and promotes growth of hepatoma cells: implications for radiotherapy of hepatocellular carcinoma. Clin Cancer Res 2006;12(9): 2706–15.

137. Camphausen KA, Lawrence RC. Principles of radiation therapy. In: Pazdur R, Wagman LD, Camphausen KA, et al, editors. Cancer management: a multidisciplinary approach. 11th edition. Lawrence (KS): CMP Healthcare Media; 2008. Available at: http://www.cancernetwork.com/cancer-management/page/1/0? gid=All&domain_id=All. Accessed October 18, 2013.

138. Tse RV, Hawkins M, Lockwood G, et al. Phase I study of individualized stereotactic body radiotherapy for hepatocellular carcinoma and intrahepatic cholangiocarcinoma. J Clin Oncol 2008;26(4):657–64.

139. Tokuuye K, Akine Y, Hashimoto T, et al. Proton beam therapy alone for hepatocellular carcinoma. Abstract 132. Presented at Gastrointestinal Cancers Symposium. Hollywood (FL), January 27–29, 2005. Meeting proceedings. 2005; p. 149.

140. Bush DA, Hillebrand DJ, Slater JM, et al. The safety and efficacy of high-dose proton beam radiotherapy for hepatocellular carcinoma: a phase 2 prospective trial. Cancer 2011;117(13):3035–59.
141. Bartolozzi C, Lencioni R, Caramella D, et al. Treatment of large HCC: transcatheter arterial chemoembolization combined with percutaneous ethanol injection versus repeated transcatheter arterial chemoembolization. Radiology 1995; 197:812–8.
142. Rossi S, Garbagnati F, Lencioni R, et al. Percutaneous radiofrequency thermal ablation of nonresectable hepatocellular carcinoma after occlusion of tumor blood supply. Radiology 2000;217:119–26.
143. Yoon S, Lim Y, Won HJ, et al. Radiotherapy plus transarterial chemoembolization for hepatocellular carcinoma invading the portal vein: long-term patient outcomes. Int J Radiat Oncol Biol Phys 2012;82:2004–11.
144. Gish RG, Porta C, Lazar L, et al. Phase III randomized controlled trial comparing the survival of patients with unresectable hepatocellular carcinoma treated with nolatrexed or doxorubicin. J Clin Oncol 2007;25:3069–75.
145. Leung TW, Patt YZ, Lau WY, et al. Complete pathological remission is possible with systemic combination chemotherapy for inoperable hepatocellular carcinoma. Clin Cancer Res 1999;5:1676–81.
146. Yeo W, Mok TS, Zee B, et al. A randomized phase III study of doxorubicin versus cisplatin/interferon alpha-2b/doxorubicin/fluorouracil (PIAF) combination chemotherapy for unresectable hepatocellular carcinoma. J Natl Cancer Inst 2005;97:1532–8.
147. Kaseb AO, Shindoh J, Patt YZ, et al. Modified cisplatin/interferon α-2b/doxorubicin/5-fluorouracil (PIAF) chemotherapy in patients with no hepatitis or cirrhosis is associated with improved response rate, resectability, and survival of initially unresectable hepatocellular carcinoma. Cancer 2013;119(18):3334–42.
148. Wilhelm SM, Carter C, Tang L, et al. BAY 43-9006 exhibits broad spectrum oral antitumor activity and targets the RAF/MEK/ERK pathway and receptor tyrosine kinases involved in tumor progression and angiogenesis. Cancer Res 2004;64: 7099–109.
149. Llovet JM, Ricci S, Mazzaferro V, et al. Sorafenib in advanced hepatocellular carcinoma. N Engl J Med 2008;359:378–90.
150. Schwartz JD, Schwartz M, Lehrer D, et al. Bevacizumab in unresectable hepatocellular carcinoma (HCC) for patients without metastasis and without invasion of the portal vein. J Clin Oncol (Meeting Abstracts) 2006;24(18S) [abstract 4144].
151. Thomas MB, Morris JS, Chadha R, et al. Phase II trial of the combination of bevacizumab and erlotinib in patients who have advanced hepatocellular carcinoma. J Clin Oncol 2009;27(6):843–50.
152. Kaseb AO, Garrett-Mayer E, Morris JS, et al. Efficacy of bevacizumab plus erlotinib for advanced hepatocellular carcinoma and predictors of outcome: final results of a phase II trial. Oncology 2012;82(2):67–74.
153. Siegel AB, Cohen EI, Ocean A, et al. Phase II trial evaluating the clinical and biologic effects of bevacizumab in unresectable hepatocellular carcinoma. J Clin Oncol 2008;26(18):2992–8.
154. Boige V, Malka D, Bourredjem A, et al. Efficacy, safety, and biomarkers of single-agent bevacizumab therapy in patients with advanced hepatocellular carcinoma. Oncologist 2012;17(8):1063–72.
155. Sun W, Haller DG, Mykulowycz K, et al. Combination of capecitabine, oxaliplatin with bevacizumab in treatment of advanced hepatocellular carcinoma (HCC): a phase II study. J Clin Oncol (Meeting Abstracts) 2007;25(18S) [abstract 4574].

156. Vogelstein B, Kinzler KW. Cancer genes and the pathways they control. Nat Med 2004;10:789–99.
157. Mendel DB, Laird AD, Xin X, et al. In vivo antitumor activity of SU11248, a novel tyrosine kinase inhibitor targeting vascular endothelial growth factor and platelet-derived growth factor receptors: determination of a pharmacokinetic/pharmacodynamic relationship. Clin Cancer Res 2003;9:327–37.
158. Hoda D, Catherine C, Strosberg J, et al. Phase II study of sunitinib malate in adult patients with metastatic or surgically unresectable hepatocellular carcinoma. Gastrointestinal Cancers Symposium, Orlando, January 25–27, 2008 (abstract 267).
159. Santoro A, Rimassa L, Borbath I, et al. Tivantinib for second-line treatment of advanced hepatocellular carcinoma: a randomised, placebo-controlled phase 2 study. Lancet Oncol 2013;14(1):55–63.
160. Morimitsu Y, Hsia CC, Kojiro M, et al. Nodules of less differentiated tumor within or adjacent to hepatocellular carcinoma: relative expression of transforming growth factor- alpha and its receptor in the different areas of tumor. Hum Pathol 1995;26:1126–32.
161. Philip PA, Mahoney MR, Allmer C, et al. Phase II study of erlotinib (OSI-774) in patients with advanced hepatocellular cancer. J Clin Oncol 2005;23:6657–63.
162. Ramanathan RK, Belani CP, Singh DA, et al. A phase II study of lapatinib in patients with advanced biliary tree and hepatocellular cancer. Cancer Chemother Pharmacol 2009;64:777–83.
163. Zhu AX, Stuart K, Blaszkowsky LS, et al. Phase 2 study of cetuximab in patients with advanced hepatocellular carcinoma. Cancer 2007;110:581–9.
164. Gruenwald V, Wilkens L, Gebel M, et al. A phase II open label study of cetuximab in unresectable hepatocellular carcinoma: final results. J Clin Oncol (Meeting Abstracts) 2007;25(18S) [abstract 4598].
165. Guo Y, Zhang Y, Klein R, et al. Irreversible electroporation therapy in the liver: longitudinal efficacy studies in a rat model of hepatocellular carcinoma. Cancer Res 2010;70:1555–63.
166. Thomas K, Chung W, Ellis S, et al. Investigation of the safety of irreversible electroporation in humans. J Vasc Interv Radiol 2011;22(5):611–21.
167. Habib N, editor. Hepatocellular carcinoma methods and protocols. Totowa (NJ): Humana Press; 2000 [Part IV. HCC gene therapy].
168. Hwang L. Gene therapy strategies for hepatocellular carcinoma. J Biomed Sc 2006;13:453–86.
169. Wu L, Pan Y, Pei X, et al. Capturing circulating tumor cells of hepatocellular carcinoma. Cancer Let 2012. http://dx.doi.org/10.1016/j.canlet.2012.07.024.
170. Xu W, Cao L, Chen L. Isolation of circulating tumor cells using a novel cell separation strategy. Clin Cancer Res 2011;17:3783–93.

Management of Antibody-Mediated Rejection in Transplantation

Basma Sadaka, PharmD, MsCR, BCPS[a], Rita R. Alloway, PharmD[a],
E. Steve Woodle, MD[b],*

KEYWORDS

- Antibody-mediated rejection • Kidney transplantation • Donor-specific antibodies
- Plasma cell

KEY POINTS

- Development of donor-specific anti-HLA antibodies following transplantation is associated with reduced allograft survival.
- To date, there are no immunosuppressive agents approved by the Food and Drug Administration to treat acute antibody-mediated rejection (AMR).
- AMR is generally less responsive then acute cellular rejection (ACR) to antirejection therapy.
- AMR is associated with lower long-term graft survival than ACR.
- Late AMR is associated with lower long-term graft survival than early AMR.
- Emerging therapies including bortezomib and eculizumab are providing promising data for managing transplant recipients who present with AMR.

INTRODUCTION

Renal allograft rejection may be T-cell mediated (acute cellular rejection [ACR]), B-cell mediated (antibody-mediated rejection [AMR]), or mixed (mixed acute rejection [MAR]). Recent studies have demonstrated that development of donor-specific anti–human leukocyte antigen (HLA) antibodies (DSA) is associated with reduced long-term graft function and survival,[1,2] and is associated with 20% to 30% of acute rejection episodes

Funding Sources: None.
Conflicts of Interest: B. Sadaka has no conflict of interest to declare. Rita R. Alloway and E. Steve Woodle have received grant funding and honoraria from Millennium Pharmaceuticals and also from Genzyme.
[a] Division of Nephrology, Department of Internal Medicine, University of Cincinnati College of Medicine, 231 Albert Sabin Way, ML 558, Cincinnati, OH 45267-0558, USA; [b] Division of Transplantation, Department of Surgery, University of Cincinnati College of Medicine, 231 Albert Sabin Way, ML 558, Cincinnati, OH 45267-0558, USA
* Corresponding author.
E-mail address: woodlees@uc.edu

Surg Clin N Am 93 (2013) 1451–1466
http://dx.doi.org/10.1016/j.suc.2013.08.002
0039-6109/13/$ – see front matter © 2013 Elsevier Inc. All rights reserved.

in kidney transplant recipients.[3,4] Despite intensive traditional immunosuppressive therapy, rates of graft loss have approximated 15% to 20% at 1 year following AMR.[3,5–7] Therefore, the development of antihumoral therapies that provide prompt elimination of DSA and improve allograft survival is an important goal.[8]

To date, there are no immunosuppressive agents approved by the Food and Drug Administration (FDA) for antibody-mediated rejection (AMR) treatment. Traditional treatment modalities for AMR include intravenous immunoglobulin (IVIg), plasmapheresis (PP), rituximab, and rabbit antithymocyte globulin (rATG). However, these agents deplete B-cell populations but not the cell at the source of antibody production, namely the mature plasma cell.[9,10] This situation has led to development of plasma cell–targeted therapies using proteasome inhibition (PI) as a novel approach for treating AMR.[11,12] This review discusses current and emerging treatment modalities used for AMR in solid organ transplantation.

DIAGNOSIS AND CLASSIFICATION OF AMR

Acute AMR diagnosis after kidney transplantation continues to undergo modifications as knowledge accumulates. The Banff '07 update remains a cornerstone for diagnosing acute AMR and includes 3 cardinal features[5,13]:

- Morphologic evidence, such as: (1) acute tissue injury and/or presence of neutrophils and/or mononuclear cells in peritubular capillaries (PTC) and/or glomeruli, (2) acute tubular injury or capillary thrombosis, and (3) intimal arteritis/fibrinoid necrosis/intramural or transmural inflammation in arteries
- Immunopathologic evidence of antibody presence, such as: (1) C4d and/or immunoglobulin in PTC or (2) immunoglobulin and complement in arterial fibrinoid necrosis
- Serologic evidence of circulating antibodies to donor HLA or DSA

Presence of C4d deposition in PTC plus 1 of the 2 criteria above leads to the diagnosis of AMR.[13]

Recently, considerable attention has focused on a variant of AMR known as C4d-negative AMR, as Halloran and colleagues[14] have emphasized the prominent importance of microcirculatory inflammation (MI). This evidence highlights the limitations of C4d, thereby suggesting that MI is likely superior to C4d as an AMR criterion.

AMR may also be classified into 3 groups based on timing: (1) hyperacute AMR, (2) acute AMR, and (3) chronic AMR.

Hyperacute AMR typically occurs within minutes to hours after allograft reperfusion and is associated with the presence of preformed antibodies against donor histocompatibility antigens. Histologic findings include neutrophil and platelet margination in glomerular and peritubular capillaritis, hemorrhagic cortical necrosis, acute tubular injury, and thrombosis and fibrin deposition within the microvasculature.

Acute AMR presents with allograft dysfunction within the first few weeks after transplantation. Major histologic findings associated with acute AMR include MI: neutrophils or mononuclear cells in the PTC or glomeruli with C4d deposition. Based on the current Banff criteria, acute AMR is classified into 3 types: type I (acute tubular necrosis), type II (glomerular type resembling thrombotic microangiopathy), and type III (vascular type with arterial inflammation). Type I represents less than 10% of patients, with only morphologic evidence of acute tubular injury with minimal tubulointerstitial neutrophil infiltrates. Type II includes peritubular capillaritis with or without glomerulitis, and type III acute AMR includes arterial inflammation with or without fibrinoid changes.

Chronic AMR clinically manifests as a slow, progressive loss of allograft function over 1 year or more after transplantation.[7,15] It is defined as having histopathologic change in addition to C4d staining in the majority of the parenchymal capillaries and small vessels, and the presence of DSA.

Of interest is subclinical AMR, a new entity described by Haas and colleagues[16] and Gloor and colleagues,[17] which was reported to be found in approximately 12% of positive DSA kidney transplant recipients undergoing desensitization, and was thought likely to contribute to chronic transplant nephropathy. Subclinical AMR meets the established pathologic and serologic criteria for AMR; however, it is not associated with graft dysfunction or concurrent ACR.[14,16–18]

AMR TREATMENT MODALITIES

Current treatment options for AMR include IVIg, PP, immunoadsorption (IA), and the administration of B-cell–targeting agents such as rituximab. A recent systematic review by Roberts and colleagues[19] addressed the treatment of acute AMR episodes in kidney transplant recipients. The purpose of the present discussion is to provide perspectives on currently used AMR treatment modalities.

Antibody Removal

Plasmapheresis

PP is the fastest and most effective method for temporary elimination of alloantibodies from the circulation. PP modalities include plasma exchange, double-filtration PP, and IA. The preferred method in the United States is plasma exchange, for reasons of cost and ease of the procedure.[20] Plasma exchange is the most commonly used method, and the term PP has been used synonymously with plasma exchange.[5] PP includes 1.0 to 1.5 plasma volume exchanges using albumin continued daily or on alternate days until serum creatinine falls within 30% of previous baseline values.[21] Between 2007 and 2010, the American Society for Apheresis upgraded its recommendation for PP in AMR from second-line to first-line therapy.[22]

Despite the efficacy of PP in removing DSA from circulation, it does not suppress antibody synthesis, and circulating DSA rebound has been documented following PP.[23] Therefore, agents that neutralize antibodies (ie, IVIg) or suppress antibody production (eg, calcineurin inhibitors, mycophenolate mofetil [MMF], rituximab, or bortezomib) are commonly used in combination with PP. Four randomized controlled trials evaluated the effect of PP in treating AMR.[24–27]

PP was reported by Kirubakaran and colleagues[24] to be potentially harmful through removal of humoral factors that may be protecting the graft. However, Bonomini and colleagues[25] reported beneficial effects with rapid removal of anti-HLA antibodies after 2 weeks of 3 to 7 daily or alternate-day PP in comparison with patients who received pharmacologic therapy alone with 2 courses of intravenous methylprednisolone × 3 days ($P<.001$). In contrast to that trial, Allen and colleagues[26] reported no effect in reduction of serum creatinine or graft survival, and concluded that PP had not been shown to modify acute renal allograft rejection. Pascual and colleagues[27] reported 100% graft survival in 5 refractory AMR patients treated with a combination of PP and rescue immunosuppression with tacrolimus and MMF at 19.6 months' mean follow-up.

Immunoadsorption

IA utilizes an adsorbent column that removes immunoglobulin G (IgG) from plasma, which is then reinfused into the patient. Replacement fluid is not needed because volume loss is minimal. IA is considered an attractive strategy as regards efficiency and highly specific antibody depletion. IA uses 1 of 2 IA columns: a protein A adsorption column that adsorbs immunoglobulin, and an ABO antigen column that adsorbs specific anti-A or anti-B antibodies regardless of immunoglobulin class or subclass.[5,28] However, IA is not commonly used to treat AMR because of cost, unavailability of the membrane, and the relative ease of PP.

Böhmig and colleagues[29] performed the only randomized controlled study of IA for AMR, which compared 5 patients in the test group who received IA (protein A columns) with another 5 patients in group B without IA with the option of IA rescue after 3 weeks. Both groups received steroid pulses plus conversion to tacrolimus/mycophenolate. Within 2 weeks, all IA-treated patients responded to treatment, whereas 4 patients in group B were dialysis dependent despite rescue IA. Min and colleagues[30] treated 6 AMR patients with IA using staphylococcal protein A plus tacrolimus/MMF, and reported 100% patient and graft survival in the IA group with an 18-month mean follow-up serum creatinine level of 1.2 mg/dL. To date there have been no studies that directly compare PP with IA in terms of efficacy and safety for AMR treatment; however, both seem to be effective.

IVIg

Immunomodulatory effects of IVIg are pleiotropic (**Fig. 1**).[31,32] IVIg enhances autoantibody clearance by blocking neonatal Fc receptors (FcRn). Continuous blockage of FcRn results in more rapid clearance of the autoantibodies.[33] IVIg also exerts neutralizing anti-idiotypic effects and blocks the action of complement.[34] Moreover, IVIg interferes with the interaction of autoimmune complexes by activating Fc γ receptors (FcγRs), and exerts negative regulatory signals via FcγRIIβ receptors.

Despite the lack of clarity in terms of the mechanism of action of IVIg, previous literature has shown that IVIg may be of benefit in AMR treatment. Luke and colleagues[35] demonstrated that IVIg rescue therapy was associated with histologic resolution or improvement of rejection severity, maintenance of renal function, and long-term graft survival for steroid-resistant and antilymphocyte-resistant rejection in renal transplant recipients. Jordan and colleagues[36] investigated the efficacy of IVIg in treating AMR in renal and cardiac transplant recipients who had no success with conventional therapies. The investigators reported that AMR resolution was noted within 2 to 5 days after IVIg administration, and all episodes of AMR were reversed, with a freedom from recurrent rejection episodes seen in 9 of 10 patients.

In 2009, Lefaucheur and colleagues[37] conducted a retrospective comparison of high-dose IVIg alone (2 g/kg administered over 2 days every 3 weeks × 4 doses) with IVIg (100 mg/kg × 4 doses and then 2 g/kg every 3 weeks × 4 doses after the last plasmapheresis session) + daily plasmapheresis (total of 4 sessions at 1.0 plasma volume exchange using 5% albumin) + rituximab 375 mg/m² (2 weekly doses after last plasmapheresis session) in patients with AMR. At 36 months, the investigators reported improved graft survival in the combined therapy group when compared with the high-dose IVIg-alone group (91.7% vs 50%, $P = .02$), as well as long-term suppression of DSA levels.

B-Cell–Specific Agents

Rituximab
Rituximab is a chimeric monoclonal anti-CD20 antibody that eliminates multiple B-cell subsets as the CD20 antigen is expressed early in B-cell ontogeny up to the point of plasma cell differentiation, where it disappears from the cell surface. The variable region of rituximab binds to CD20 and marks the cell for destruction by apoptosis, complement-dependent cytotoxicity, and/or antibody-dependent cell-mediated

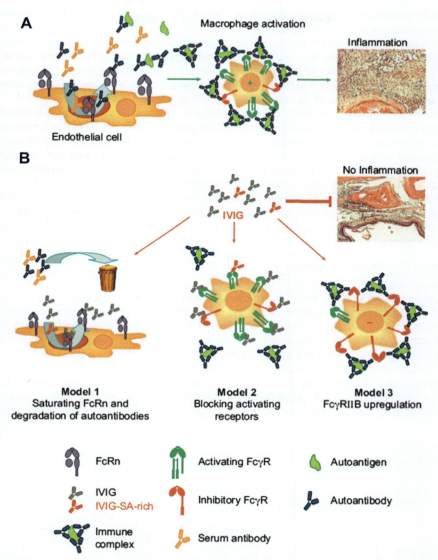

Fig. 1. Immunomodulatory effects of intravenous immunoglobulin. (*A*) The neonatal Fc receptor (FcRn) binds to serum IgG at low pH after it has been endocytosed and transported into acidic vesicles. FcRn-bound IgG molecules are then recycled to the cell surface and released into the circulation at physiologic pH. (*B*) Three different models have been proposed to mediate the anti-inflammatory activity of the IVIG Fc fragment in vivo. First, the high dose of IgG molecules present in the IVIG preparation may compete with autoantibodies for FcRn binding and thus result in their enhanced clearance. Second, immune complexes present in the IVIG preparation may bind to activating FcγRs and thereby prevent binding of autoantibody immune complexes. In the third model, IVIG activity is crucially dependent on the presence of the inhibitory FcγRIIB. (*From* Nimmerjahn F, Ravetch JV. Anti-inflammatory actions of intravenous immunoglobulin. Annu Rev Immunol 2008;26:520; with permission.)

cellular cytotoxicity. Apoptosis occurs as a result of the activation of caspases by the cross-linking of bound CD20 proteins.[38,39]

Becker and colleagues[40] conducted an initial report on the benefit of using rituximab in treating refractory rejection in 27 patients who had received treatment with steroids, plasmapheresis, and/or rATG without improvement in creatinine. Overall, 24 patients had good allograft function at the time of discharge, and 3 patients had graft loss after receiving a single dose of rituximab (375 mg/m²) as salvage therapy.

Fifty-four patients with AMR were evaluated in a retrospective 2-year outcomes study by Kaposztas and colleagues.[41] Of these patients, 26 received plasmapheresis and rituximab, and 28 received plasmapheresis without rituximab. Patients who presented with low serum IgG levels also received IVIg. Two-year graft survival was significantly better in the rituximab group (90% vs 60%), and a trend toward improved graft survival was also seen in those patients who had received IVIg ($P = .0052$).

Mulley and colleagues[42] reported a case series of 7 patients with refractory AMR who responded to treatment with 1 dose of rituximab (500 mg). Recovery of kidney function with 100% graft survival was reported in all patients after a mean follow-up of 21 months.

Plasma Cell–Depleting Agents

Bortezomib

Bortezomib (Millennium Pharmaceuticals, Cambridge, MA) is a first-in-class proteasome inhibitor originally approved by the FDA for the treatment of multiple myeloma in 2003.[43] The efficacy of bortezomib was first demonstrated in the treatment of refractory AMR in renal transplant recipients,[11] and was subsequently shown to provide effective primary therapy for AMR.[12]

The 26S proteasome is a multimeric complex that consists of a 20S core and 1 or 2 19S regulatory particles (**Fig. 2**).[6,44–47] The normal physiologic role of the proteasome is to degrade misfolded proteins into peptides. Misfolded proteins are ubiquitin labeled, which targets them for proteasome degradation.[46] Inhibition of proteasome

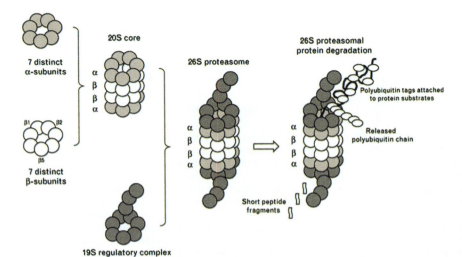

Fig. 2. The 26S proteasome and ubiquitin-mediated protein degradation. (*From* Everly JJ, Walsh RC, Alloway RR, et al. Proteasome inhibition for antibody-mediated rejection. Curr Opin Organ Transplant 2009;14(6):663; with permission.)

activity results in profound biochemical and physiologic events. Induction of stress on the endoplasmic reticulum, which may culminate in programmed cell death, is thought to be a major mechanism of action of proteasome inhibitors on myeloma cells and normal plasma cells.[44,46] Other important effects of proteasome inhibitors include inhibition of nuclear factor κB activation, cell-cycle arrest-induced programmed cell death, caspase activation, and inhibition of major histocompatibility complex class I–restricted antigen presentation.[6,44–47]

Recent clinical experiences have described the effects of bortezomib in AMR. The first report of bortezomib use in renal transplantation included 8 MAR episodes (both AMR and ACR components and defined as biopsy-proven acute rejection meeting Banff '97 criteria) in 6 transplant recipients found to be refractory to plasmapheresis, IVIg, ± rATG, ± rituximab.[11] Each cycle of bortezomib consisted of 4 doses at 1.3 mg/m^2, which was similar to the dosing used to treat patients with multiple myeloma. Despite these refractory rejection episodes, MAR was reversed after bortezomib treatment. Renal function improved or remained stable, and resolution or improvement was noted on the posttreatment biopsies. In addition to the improvement in renal allograft survival, the immunodominant DSA (iDSA), defined as the DSA with the highest levels, were decreased by more than 50% within 14 days and remained substantially suppressed for up to 5 months.[11] Perry and colleagues[10] subsequently described bortezomib therapy in 2 kidney transplant recipients with AMR, and showed a decrease in bone marrow plasma cells that produced DSA.

Primary bortezomib therapy for antibody-mediated renal allograft rejection was described by Walsh and colleagues.[12] The PI-based regimen consisted of 4 doses of bortezomib (1.3 mg/m^2) with plasmapheresis sessions immediately before each dose of bortezomib, and 1 dose of rituximab (375 mg/m^2) administered with the first dose of bortezomib only. Before each PP session, DSA samples were collected using single-antigen beads on a Luminex platform. Two patients presented with high DSA levels and positive peritubular or glomerular C4d staining consisting with acute AMR and occurring within the first 2 weeks after transplantation. After administration of the PI regimen, both patients experienced prompt reversal of their AMR episodes and elimination of DSA within 14 days of therapy. One patient required a second cycle of bortezomib after 2 months of initial therapy owing to repeated elevation of DSA, including 2 new HLA specificities, and prompt DSA elimination was established.[12]

Variations in clinical response to PI therapy were noted and experienced by comparison of results in early and late AMR.[48] Late AMR, which was defined as occurring 6 months after transplantation, has been long known to be associated with poor graft outcome.[49,50] In the analysis by Walsh and colleagues,[48] 17 patients who presented with late AMR and 13 with early AMR were compared. Higher iDSA levels were more prevalent in the late AMR patients than in the early AMR group, and specificities were primarily class II (DQ being most frequent). Greater reduction in iDSA levels at 7 days, 14 days, 30 days, and posttreatment nadir were reported in the early AMR patients (81.5% ± 21.2% vs 51.4% ± 27.6%; $P<.01$). Both groups demonstrated significant improvement in renal function; however, early AMR patients were more likely to demonstrate histologic improvement on repeat biopsy.[48]

Recently published results by Dörje and colleagues[51] were consistent with those reported by Walsh and colleagues.[48] In this analysis, kidney recipients were stratified by early AMR (n = 40) and late AMR (n = 27). Early AMR was defined as an AMR episode occurring less than 3 months after transplantation, with late AMR occurring later than 3 months after transplantation. Recipients with late AMR had significantly reduced graft survival in comparison with those presenting with early AMR ($P<.001$, log-rank test; 40% vs 75% at 4 years; hazard ratio 3.72; 95% confidence interval

1.65–8.42).[51] Of interest, the investigators concluded that the late AMR group was characterized by younger recipient age (37.9 ± 12 vs 50.9 ± 11.6 years; $P<.001$), increased occurrence of de novo DSA (52% vs 13%; $P = .001$), and nonadherence/suboptimal immunosuppression (56% vs 0%; $P<.001$).[51]

Flechner and colleagues[52] reported their experience with bortezomib coadministered with IVIg in treating 16 kidney-only and 4 kidney-combined organ recipients presenting with DSA and histologic evidence of AMR diagnosed approximately 20 months after transplantation (range 1–71 months).[52] Patients received intravenous corticosteroids followed by a 2-week cycle of PP and 1.3 mg/m² of bortezomib on days 1, 4, 8, and 11, then IVIg 0.5 mg/kg.[52] This experience suggested that those who have significant AMR may respond less to a bortezomib-based regimen because of the reduced therapeutic response in patients with significant renal dysfunction.

In terms of the safety profile of bortezomib, Schmidt and colleagues[53] reported that minimal toxicity resulted from the use of bortezomib in both AMR patients and desensitization candidates. Similar degrees and incidence of bone marrow suppression, gastrointestinal side effects, and peripheral neuropathy were demonstrated in comparison with the toxicity profile in the multiple myeloma population. The National Cancer Institute Common Terminology Criteria for Adverse Events was used to grade hematologic toxicities (neutropenia, anemia, and thrombocytopenia) and gastrointestinal toxicities (nausea, vomiting, and diarrhea). Peripheral neuropathy was gauged by the administration of the Peripheral Neuropathy Scale adapted from the Gynecologic Oncology Group, and graded based on duration and severity of symptoms.[54] Only anemia and peripheral neuropathy were noted to be significant toxicities after bortezomib use; however, they were manageable (**Table 1**).[53] All other toxicities occurred at a lower or similar frequency to that in the multiple myeloma group (**Table 2**).[53,55,56]

Complement-Specific Agents

The complement cascade was first described by Ehrlich in the late 1890s and was subsequently characterized by Bordet; however, the role of complement factors in the immune response to organ transplantation has been extensively studied only in recent years.[57]

A major mechanism of antibody-mediated injury in kidney transplant recipients is thought to be the activation of the complement cascade by DSA (**Fig. 3**),[57] resulting in direct injury, and also the enhancement of cellular infiltration and inflammation in the allograft. Therefore, the use of agents that cause blockade of complement component C5 may reduce the incidence of early AMR in sensitized renal transplant recipients, making this concept an intriguing therapeutic modality in preventing and treating early graft loss.[57]

Eculizumab

Eculizumab (Soliris; Alexion, Cheshire, CT, USA) is a humanized monoclonal antibody with a high binding affinity for the C5 protein of the complement activation cascade through the C3 convertase molecules (see **Fig. 3**).[57,58] The result of this inhibition leads to prevention of the formation of the C5b-C9 membrane attack complex. Initially, eculizumab received FDA approval for the treatment of paroxysmal nocturnal hemoglobinuria[59]; however, because of its role in the complement system, further studies have been conducted to evaluate its important role in other immunologic disorders that involve complement activation.

To date, eculizumab use in transplantation has been reported through limited case reports as salvage therapy for severe episodes of AMR. Locke and colleagues[60] reported their success with one patient on the use of eculizumab (in combination

Table 1
Bortezomib toxicity data and incidence

	AMR (n = 51)	Desensitization (n = 19)	P value
Baseline hemoglobin (Hgb) (g/dL)	10.2 ± 1.5	12.7 ± 1.8	<.0001
Hgb at nadir (g/dL)	7.9 ± 1.7	11.3 ± 2.1	<.0001
CTCAE Grade 2 Anemia (%)	26.2	20.0	NS
CTCAE Grade 3 Anemia (%)	39.3	2.9	.002
CTCAE Grade 4 Anemia (%)	16.4	0	.0130
Baseline platelets (10^3 cells/mm^3)	220.4 ± 78.2	211.6 ± 85.2	NS
Platelets at nadir (10^3 cells/mm^3)	108.2 ± 53.9	113.0 ± 55.0	NS
CTCAE Grade 1 Thrombocytopenia (%)	13.1	14.3	NS
CTCAE Grade 3 Thrombocytopenia (%)	11.5	8.6	NS
CTCAE Grade 4 Thrombocytopenia (%)	3.3	0	NS
Baseline ANC (cells/mm^3 × 1000) (%)	7.0 ± 3.7	3.8 ± 1.8	<.0001
ANC at nadir (cells/mm^3)	3.3 ± 2.1	3.1 ± 1.4	NS
CTCAE Grade 2 Neutropenia (%)	6.6	0	NS
CTCAE Grade 3 Neutropenia (%)	4.9	2.9	NS
CTCAE Grade 4 Neutropenia (%)	3.3	0	NS
Baseline peripheral neuropathy [PN] (%)	17.0	36.8	NS
Worsening of baseline PN (%)	22.2	57.1	NS
New-onset Bortezomib-induced PN [BIPN] (%)	27.3	58.3	.0494
BIPN Level 1 or 2 (%)	15.1	31.6	NS
BIPN Level 3 (%)	3.8	21.1	.0223
BIPN Level 4 (%)	5.7	0	NS
BIPN Level 5 (%)	1.9	5.3	NS

Abbreviations: AMR, Antibody-mediated rejection; ANC, Absolute neutrophil counts; BIPN, Bortezomib-induced peripheral neuropathy; CTCAE, Common terminology criteria for adverse events; Hgb, Hemoglobin; NS, Not significant; PN, Peripheral neuropathy.

From Schmidt N, Alloway RR, Walsh RC, et al. Prospective evaluation of the toxicity profile of proteasome inhibitor-based therapy in renal transplant candidates and recipients. Transplantation 2012;94(4):352–61; with permission.

with plasmapheresis/IVIg) in an episode of severe antibody-mediated renal allograft rejection presented at postoperative day 9. Three days after eculizumab administration, urine output returned and the patient recovered from AMR with a serum creatinine returning to 1.1 mg/dL.

Stegall and colleagues[61] compared AMR incidence within 3 months after transplantation between a historical group of patients that did not receive any eculizumab and a group that consisted of 26 highly sensitized kidney transplant recipients. The investigators reported a markedly decreased incidence of AMR in the eculizumab group when compared with the control group (7.7% vs 41.2%).[61]

AMR Rescue by Splenectomy

Splenectomy provides a seldom used option to salvage kidney allografts from severe acute AMR that is unresponsive to conventional AMR treatment.

Locke and colleagues[62] published their results with rescue splenectomy in 5 highly sensitized patients with refractory AMR. Resolution of histologic signs of AMR and functioning grafts was reported in all patients and after a mean follow-up of

Table 2
Bortezomib toxicities: comparison between transplant and multiple myeloma populations

	Grade 3				Grade 4			
	AMR	DS	Richardson,[55] et al	Orlowski,[56] et al	AMR	DS	Richardson,[11] et al	Orlowski,[12] et al
Diarrhea, %	0	0	7	4	0	0	0	0
Nausea, %	0	0	2	<1	0	0	0	0
Vomiting, %	0	0	3	1	0	0	0	0
Peripheral neuropathy, %	5.7	0	7	9[a]	1.9	5.3	1	9[a]
Thrombocytopenia, %	11.5	8.6	26	8	3.3	0	4	8
Anemia, %	39.3	2.9	9	7	16.4	0	1	2
Neutropenia, %	4.9	2.9	12	11	3.3	0	2	4

Abbreviations: AMR, antibody-mediated rejection; DS, desensitization.

[a] Includes both grades 3 and 4 peripheral neuropathy.

From Schmidt N, Alloway RR, Walsh RC, et al. Prospective evaluation of the toxicity profile of proteasome inhibitor-based therapy in renal transplant candidates and recipients. Transplantation 2012;94(4):352–61; with permission.

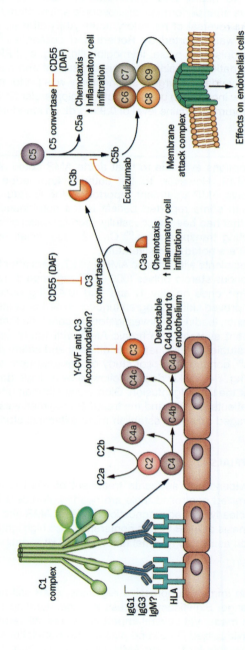

Fig. 3. Role of the complement pathway and eculizumab target in AMR. (*From* Stegall MD, Chedid MF, Cornell LD. The role of complement in antibody-mediated rejection in kidney transplantation. Nat Rev Nephrol 2012;8:672; with permission.)

18 months. Kaplan and colleagues[63] reported results with rescue splenectomy in refractory AMR with immediate improvement in urinary output, reduction in serum
creatinine levels within 48 hours, and conversion of ABO-incompatible patient
cross-matches to negative after performing laparoscopic splenectomy in 4 refractory
AMR patients. Successful reversal of refractory acute AMR after splenectomy in a
highly sensitized patient was reported by Roberti and colleagues.[64] The patient
was started on methylprednisolone pulse, thymoglobulin, IVIg, and PP; however, by
postoperative day 14 the patient remained dialysis dependent and had no response
to therapy. By postoperative day 14, urgent splenectomy was performed and the investigators reported a slow increase in urine output and glomerular filtration rate, with
a 1-year posttransplant serum creatinine level of 0.9 mg/dL on standard maintenance
immunosuppression.[64]

Chronic AMR Treatment

In theory, all treatment options available to treat acute AMR could also be used in
patients with chronic AMR. However, to the authors' knowledge there are no
controlled trials for chronic AMR treatment reported in the literature to date. The
only treatment option with some reported benefit is the combination of rituximab
and IVIg, a combination that had been successfully used for desensitization of highly
sensitized patients awaiting transplantation.[65] Only 2 case series on treatment of
established chronic AMR are noted in the literature.

Four kidney allograft recipients with chronic AMR 1 to 27 years after transplantation
were treated with intravenous steroid pulses (500–1000 mg once daily for 3–5 days),
and rituximab (375 mg/m^2 once on day 1) and IVIg (0.4 g/kg once daily on day
2–5).[66] Rituximab/IVIg improved kidney allograft function in all 4 patients, with a reduction in DSA in 2 of 4 patients, leading the investigators to conclude that rituximab/IVIg
may be a useful treatment strategy for chronic AMR with future establishment of
randomized multicenter studies for evaluating its efficacy and safety profile.[66]

Billing and colleagues[67] conducted a pilot study on the treatment of chronic AMR
with high-dose IVIg (1 g/kg × 4 weekly doses), followed by a single dose of rituximab
(375 mg/m^2) 1 week after the last IVIg infusion. Glomerular filtration rates improved or
stabilized in 4 of the 6 patients ($P<.05$), and the treatment regimen was well tolerated.
This observation encouraged others to establish more extensive studies to evaluate
this treatment strategy.

FUTURE AMR CLINICAL TRIALS

The current available evidence on adequate treatment of AMR is insufficient and
prospective, and randomized controlled trials are needed. A recent FDA workshop
highlighted the need for clearly defined diagnostic criteria for AMR and a better understanding of the pathogenesis of AMR.[68] This conference also highlighted the need for
validated end points such as histology, renal function, and HLA-antibody levels.

SUMMARY

Despite improvements in immunosuppressive regimens, AMR still remains a significant therapeutic challenge. Significant progress in understanding the pathophysiology of AMR has been made, yet several important issues still remain unresolved,
including the role of individualized B-cell and plasma-cell populations.

Several agents are available for treating AMR, including: (1) IVIg, (2) PP, (3) rituximab, (4) rATG, (5) bortezomib, and (6) eculizumab; however, clinical development of
these agents will require advancement in the end points of clinical trial designs.

Preliminary evidence of successfully treating and preventing AMR with new agents is encouraging; however, larger, randomized controlled trials with long-term follow-up are required to determine whether these advances actually improve outcomes of AMR.

REFERENCES

1. Mao Q, Terasaki PI, Cai J, et al. Extremely high association between appearance of HLA antibodies and failure of kidney grafts in a five-year longitudinal study. Am J Transplant 2007;7:864–71.
2. Lee PC, Zhu L, Terasaki PI, et al. HLA-specific antibodies developed in the first year posttransplant are predictive of chronic rejection and renal graft loss. Transplantation 2009;88:568–74.
3. Mauiyyedi S, Colvin RB. Humoral rejection in kidney transplantation: new concepts in diagnosis and treatment. Curr Opin Nephrol Hypertens 2002;11:609–18.
4. Lederer SR, Friedrich N, Banas B, et al. Effects of mycophenolate mofetil on donor-specific antibody formation in renal transplantation. Clin Transplant 2005;19(2):168–74.
5. Lucas JG, Co JP, Nwaogwugwu UT, et al. Antibody-mediated rejection in kidney transplantation: an update. Expert Opin Pharmacother 2011;12(4):579–92.
6. Sadaka B, Alloway RR, Woodle ES. Clinical and investigational use of proteasome inhibitors for transplant rejection. Expert Opin Investig Drugs 2011; 20(11):1535–42.
7. Takemoto SK, Zeevi A, Feng S, et al. National conference to assess antibody-mediated rejection in solid organ transplantation. Am J Transplant 2004;4:1033–41.
8. Everly MJ, Everly JJ, Arend LJ, et al. Reducing de novo donor-specific antibody levels during acute rejection diminishes renal allograft loss. Am J Transplant 2009;9:1063–71.
9. Ramos EJ, Pollinger HS, Stegall MD, et al. The effect of desensitization protocols on human splenic B-cell populations in vivo. Am J Transplant 2007;7:402–7.
10. Perry DK, Burns JM, Pollinger HS, et al. Proteasome inhibition causes apoptosis of normal human plasma cells preventing alloantibody production. Am J Transplant 2009;9:201–9.
11. Everly MJ, Everly JJ, Susskind B, et al. Bortezomib provides effective therapy for antibody- and cell-mediated acute rejection. Transplantation 2008;86:1754–61.
12. Walsh RC, Everly JJ, Brailey P, et al. Proteasome inhibitor-based primary therapy for antibody-mediated renal allograft rejection. Transplantation 2010;89: 277–84.
13. Solez K, Colvin RB, Racusen LC, et al. Banff 07 classification of renal allograft pathology: updates and future directions. Am J Transplant 2008;8:753–60.
14. Halloran PF, de Freitas DG, Einecke G, et al. An integrated view of molecular changes, histopathology and outcomes in kidney transplants. Am J Transplant 2010;10(10):2223–30.
15. Colvin RB. Pathology of chronic humoral rejection. Contrib Nephrol 2009;162: 75–86.
16. Haas M, Montgomery RA, Segave DL, et al. Subclinical acute antibody-mediated rejection in positive crossmatch renal allografts. Am J Transplant 2007;7:576–85.
17. Gloor JM, Cosio FG, Rea DJ, et al. Histologic findings one year after positive crossmatch or ABO blood group incompatible living donor kidney transplantation. Am J Transplant 2006;6:1841–7.

18. Loupy A, Suberbielle-Boissel C, Hill GS, et al. Outcome of subclinical antibody-mediated rejection in kidney transplant recipients with preformed donor-specific antibodies. Am J Transplant 2009;9:2561–70.
19. Roberts DM, Jian SH, Chadban SJ. The treatment of acute antibody-mediated rejection in kidney transplant recipients—a systematic review. Transplantation 2012;94:775–83.
20. Singh N, Pirsch J, Samaniego M. Antibody mediated rejection: treatment alternatives and outcome. Transplant Rev (Orlando) 2009;23(1):34–46.
21. Sureshkumar KK, Hussain SM, Carpenter BJ, et al. Antibody-mediated rejection following renal transplantation. Expert Opin Pharmacother 2007;8(7):913–21.
22. Ahmed T, Senzel L. The role of therapeutic apheresis in the treatment of acute antibody-mediated kidney rejection. J Clin Apher 2012;27(4):173–7.
23. Rocha PN, Butterly DW, Greenberg A, et al. Beneficial effect of plasmapheresis and intravenous immunoglobulin on renal allograft survival of patients with acute humoral rejection. Transplantation 2003;75(9):1490–5.
24. Kirubakaran MG, Disney AP, Norman J, et al. A controlled trial of plasmapheresis in the treatment of renal allograft rejection. Transplantation 1981;32(2):164–5.
25. Bonomini V, Vangelista A, Frasca GM, et al. Effects of plasmapheresis in renal transplant rejection. A controlled study. Trans Am Soc Artif Intern Organs 1985;31:698–703.
26. Allen NH, Dyer P, Geoghegan T, et al. Plasma exchange in acute renal allograft rejection. A controlled trial. Transplantation 1983;35(5):425–8.
27. Pascual M, Saidman S, Tolkoff-Rubin N, et al. Plasma exchange and tacrolimus-mycophenolate rescue for acute humoral rejection in kidney transplantation. Transplantation 1998;66:1460–4.
28. Tyden G, Kumlien G, Efvergren M. Present techniques for antibody removal. Transplantation 2007;84:S27–9.
29. Böhmig GA, Wahrmann M, Reagele H, et al. Immunoadsorption in severe C4d-positive acute kidney allograft rejection: a randomized controlled trial. Am J Transplant 2007;7(1):117–21.
30. Min L, Shuming G, Zheng T, et al. Novel rescue therapy for C4d-positive acute humoral renal allograft rejection. Clin Transplant 2005;19(1):51–5.
31. Kihm LP, Zeier M, Morath C. Emerging drugs for the treatment of transplant rejection. Expert Opin Emerg Drugs 2011;16(4):683–95.
32. Kazatchkine MD, Kaveri SV. Immunomodulation of autoimmune and inflammatory diseases with intravenous immune globulin. N Engl J Med 2001;345:747–55.
33. Nimmerjahn F, Ravetch JV. Anti-inflammatory actions of intravenous immunoglobulin. Annu Rev Immunol 2008;26:513–33.
34. Vani J, Elluru S, Negi V, et al. Role of natural antibodies in immune homeostasis: IVIg perspective. Autoimmun Rev 2008;7(6):440–4.
35. Luke PP, Scantlebury VP, Jordan ML, et al. IVIG rescue therapy in renal transplantation. Transplant Proc 2001;33:1093–4.
36. Jordan S, Quartel AW, Czer LS, et al. Posttransplant therapy using high-dose human immunoglobulin (intravenous gammaglobulin) to control acute humoral rejection in renal and cardiac allograft recipients and potential mechanism of action. Transplantation 1998;66(6):800–5.
37. Lefaucheur C, Nochy D, Andrade J, et al. Comparison of combination plasmapheresis/IVIg/anti-CD20 versus high-dose IVIg in the treatment of antibody-mediated rejection. Am J Transplant 2009;9(5):1099–107.

38. Clynes RA, Towers TL, Presta LG, et al. Inhibitory Fc receptors modulate in vivo cytotoxicity against tumor targets. Nat Med 2000;6:443–6.
39. Weiner GJ. Rituximab: mechanism of action. Semin Hematol 2010;47:115–23.
40. Becker YT, Becker BN, Pirsch JD, et al. Rituximab as treatment for refractory kidney transplant rejection. Am J Transplant 2004;4:996–1001.
41. Kaposztas Z, Podder H, Mauiyyedi S, et al. Impact of rituximab therapy for treatment of acute humoral rejection. Clin Transplant 2009;23:63–73.
42. Mulley WR, Hudson FJ, Tait BD, et al. A single low-fixed dose of rituximab to salvage renal transplants from refractory antibody-mediated rejection. Transplantation 2009;87:286–9.
43. Velcade [package insert]. Cambridge, MA: Millennium Pharmaceuticals, Inc; 2013.
44. Everly JJ, Walsh RC, Alloway RR, et al. Proteasome inhibition for antibody-mediated rejection. Curr Opin Organ Transplant 2009;14:662–6.
45. Kloetzel PM, Ossendorp F. Proteasome and peptidase function in MHC-class I-mediated antigen presentation. Curr Opin Immunol 2004;16:76–81.
46. Kim R, Emi M, Tanabe K, et al. Role of the unfolded protein response in cell death. Apoptosis 2006;11:5–13.
47. Adams J. The proteasome: structure, function, and role in the cell. Cancer Treat Rev 2003;29(Suppl 1):3–9.
48. Walsh RC, Brailey P, Girnita A, et al. Early and late acute antibody-mediated rejection differs immunologically and in response to proteasome inhibition. Transplantation 2011;91(11):1218–26.
49. Basadonna GP, Matas AJ, Gillingham KJ, et al. Early versus late acute renal allograft rejection: impact on chronic rejection. Transplantation 1993;55:993–5.
50. Sipkens YW, Doxidis II, Mallat MJ, et al. Early versus late acute rejection episodes in renal transplantation. Transplantation 2004;75:204–8.
51. Dörje C, Midtvedt K, Holdaas H, et al. Early versus late acute antibody-mediated rejection in renal transplant recipients. Transplantation 2013;96(1):79–84.
52. Flechner SM, Fatica R, Askar M, et al. The role of proteasome inhibition with bortezomib in the treatment of antibody-mediated rejection after kidney-only or kidney-combined organ transplantation. Transplantation 2010;90:1486–92.
53. Schmidt N, Alloway RR, Walsh RC, et al. Prospective evaluation of the toxicity profile of proteasome inhibitor-based therapy in renal transplant candidates and recipients. Transplantation 2012;94(4):352–61.
54. Almadrones L, McGuire DB, Walczak JR, et al. Psychometric evaluation of two scales assessing functional status and peripheral neuropathy associated with chemotherapy for ovarian cancer: a gynecologic oncology group study. Oncol Nurs Forum 2004;31(3):615–23.
55. Richardson PG, Sonneveld P, Schuster MW, et al. Bortezomib or high-dose dexamethasone for relapsed multiple myeloma. N Engl J Med 2005;352(24):2487–98.
56. Orlowski RZ, Nagler A, Sonneveld P, et al. Randomized phase III study of pegylated liposomal doxorubicin plus bortezomib compared with bortezomib alone in relapsed or refractory multiple myeloma: combination therapy improves time to progression. J Clin Oncol 2007;25(25):3892–901.
57. Stegall MD, Chedid MF, Cornell LD. The role of complement in antibody-mediated rejection in kidney transplantation. Nat Rev Nephrol 2012;8:670–8.
58. González-Roncero F, Suñer M, Bernal G, et al. Eculizumab treatment of acute antibody-mediated rejection in renal transplantation: case reports. Transplant Proc 2012;44:2690–4.

59. Hillmen P, Young NS, Schubert J, et al. The complement inhibitor eculizumab in paroxysmal nocturnal hemoglobinuria. N Engl J Med 2006;355:1233–43.
60. Locke JE, Magro CM, Singer AL, et al. The use of antibody to complement protein C5 for salvage treatment of severe antibody-mediated rejection. Am J Transplant 2009;9:231–5.
61. Stegall MD, Diwan T, Raghavaiah S, et al. Terminal complement inhibition decreases antibody-mediated rejection in sensitized renal transplant recipients. Am J Transplant 2011;11:2405–13.
62. Locke JE, Zachary AA, Haas M, et al. The utility of splenectomy as rescue treatment for severe acute antibody mediated rejection. Am J Transplant 2007;7: 842–6.
63. Kaplan B, Gangemi A, Thielke J, et al. Successful rescue of refractory, severe antibody mediated rejection with splenectomy. Transplantation 2007;83(1): 99–100.
64. Roberti I, Geffner S, Vyas S. Successful rescue of refractory acute antibody-mediated renal allograft rejection with splenectomy—a case report. Pediatr Transplant 2012;16(2):E49–52.
65. Vo AA, Lukovsky M, Toyoda M, et al. Rituximab and intravenous immune globulin for desensitization during renal transplantation. N Engl J Med 2008;359: 242–51.
66. Fehr T, Rusi B, Fischer A, et al. Rituximab and intravenous immunoglobulin treatment of chronic antibody-mediated kidney allograft rejection. Transplantation 2009;87(12):1837–41.
67. Billing H, Rieger S, Ovens J, et al. Successful treatment of chronic antibody-mediated rejection with IVIg and rituximab in pediatric renal transplant recipients. Transplantation 2008;86(9):1214–21.
68. Archdeacon P, Chan M, Neuland C, et al. Summary of FDA antibody-mediated rejection workshop. Am J Transplant 2011;11:896–906.

The Transplant Center and Business Unit as a Model for Specialized Care Delivery

A. Osama Gaber, MD[a,b,c,*], Roberta L. Schwartz, MHS[b],
David P. Bernard, MBA/MHA[b,c], Susan Zylicz, RN, BSN, MBA[c]

KEYWORDS

- Transplant center • Business unit • Transplantation health care delivery
- Transplantation

KEY POINTS

- Transplantation is one of the most regulated fields in medicine. This extensive regulatory oversight has evolved from the reliance of the transplantation effort on governmental resources and public trust to maintain the voluntary system of organ donation and from the expanded role of public payment for transplantation through the Medicare program.
- Transplantation is a hospital-based service. Medicare reimburses hospitals for the costs of pretransplant evaluation and listing of Medicare patients.
- Defining the area of focus or mission of a transplant center is crucial to the alignment of the function of the physicians and health care providers performing the clinical functions. Defining the mission of the transplant business unit is also crucial to the ability of the organization to plan for the needed resources and for the expected outcomes from the transplant effort.
- Integrating the care of patients with organ failure in the transplant center allows the organization to fully assimilate the business development, marketing, and public awareness campaigns needed to grow and sustain the center and, thus, to best serve bigger groups of its patients.
- It is imperative that a transplant center, as a patient-focused enterprise, must have a set of clinical patient-centered outcomes at the core of its scorecard. The results can be assessed by comparing the outcomes with the expected norms, such as those published by the Scientific Registry of Transplantation or the University Hospital Consortium, or to other benchmarks that are developed locally in areas where no published measures exist.

Presented in part at the ATC Annual Meeting. Boston, May 30-June 3, 2009.
[a] Department of Surgery, Houston Methodist Hospital, 6550 Fannin Street, Smith Tower 1661, Houston, TX 77030, USA; [b] Houston Methodist Hospital, Houston, TX, USA; [c] Methodist J.C. Walter Transplant Center, Houston Methodist Hospital, Houston, TX, USA
* Corresponding author. Department of Surgery, Houston Methodist Hospital, 6550 Fannin Street, Smith Tower 1661, Houston, TX 77030.
E-mail address: aogaber@houstonmethodist.org

Surg Clin N Am 93 (2013) 1467–1477
http://dx.doi.org/10.1016/j.suc.2013.08.005
0039-6109/13/$ – see front matter © 2013 Elsevier Inc. All rights reserved.

surgical.theclinics.com

INTRODUCTION

Over the past half century, transplantation has evolved from an experimental discipline into a more mature, clinical discipline. Significant advances in transplantation medicine and research have fueled this evolution. Transplant centers are not only a valuable asset to a transplantation hospital but are also essential to organize the delivery of care to patients with diseases that cause organ failure. A well-designed transplant center drives better clinical results through an administrative organization that streamlines patient care and aspires to achieve the best clinical outcomes. Through continuous monitoring of clinical and financial outcomes, the transplant center allows the organization to achieve an appropriate and rapid response to the changing landscape of health care. This article seeks to explain what sets the transplant center apart from other methods of organization, focusing on how a well-administered center suits the needs of a burgeoning transplantation program.

Transplantation is unique among other medical disciplines because of its unparalleled reliance on public support and trust through organ donation[1–3] and on governmental funding through direct payments from Medicare and Medicaid programs for a significant proportion of transplant procedures[4] and through the Medicare payments to hospitals for transplant costs as part of the hospital cost report. Additionally, because of its high costs, transplantation payers have much more structured payment schemes and performance-based contracting.[5] These unique aspects of the discipline influence the structure, function, and oversight of transplantation and define the business of delivering care through a transplant center.

TRANSPLANTATION AS A HOSPITAL-BASED SERVICE: FINANCES AND THE COST REPORT

Transplantation is a hospital-based service. Medicare reimburses hospitals for costs of pretransplant evaluation and listing of Medicare patients. In addition, Medicare reimburses hospitals for all costs incurred for acquiring organs for transplantation. These organ costs are paid by the hospital to the organ procurement organizations for cadaveric organs. For living donors, the hospital accumulates costs of evaluation of living donors and all costs related to kidney or other organ excision, including costs of donor postoperative follow-up and treatment of donation-related complications for up to 2 years. These organ-acquisition costs are passed through to the Medicare cost report. Medicare reimburses the hospitals for a portion of the costs (ie, all costs incurred by Medicare beneficiaries by calculating the percent of kidneys and or other organs transplanted into Medicare beneficiaries).[6] This organizational scheme allows the hospitals to staff their pretransplant centers and to perform an adequate workup on potential donors and recipients. Because private payers bundle organ acquisition into the transplant contracts, the hospitals have an incentive to maintain the overall costs in check because escalating costs render non-Medicare organs too expensive and noncompetitive for private insurance.[7]

Posttransplant costs are paid to the hospitals by Medicare through diagnosis-related grouping (DRG) payments (part A payments). Each type of organ transplant is assigned a DRG based on its complexity. The hospital reimbursement for each DRG is determined by a formula that takes into account the DRG weight, the amount of resource utilization in the care, a national standardized amount, and the local wage index. Each transplant DRG is based on an expected length of stay for each diagnosis.[8] Most transplant DRGs have modifiers to indicate the case complexity and comorbid condition, with the notable exception of the kidney DRG. Once patients are discharged and are readmitted after a certain time, a new and different DRG is assigned to the new admission with a new diagnosis and new payment.[9] DRG payments are subject to denial based on medical necessity, so that a readmission to the hospital has to be justified by the severity of illness or complexity of the intervention needed. Unlike private payers, Medicare does not generally require prior authorization for readmissions; but payments are subject to review and can be withheld or recouped based on postreview.[10] Medicare has designed a system for paying for exceptionally expensive cases. The methodology involves calculating a fixed loss amount per DRG (approximately $42 000 for kidney transplant) after which Medicare would pay a percent of the hospital charges. Various insurance and private payers contract with hospitals for bundled care in which an individual payment is issued for the transplant admission and a certain amount of postoperative care. The hospital is usually at risk for cases that are more costly than the contracted amount until a certain threshold of days of care or dollar amount is reached. After hitting any of these stop-loss parameters, the payer starts reimbursing the outlier costs, usually as a percent of the charges. These arrangements align the hospital's and the private payer's interests in decreasing the cost of care and cap the potential financial exposure of the payers except for the outlier cases that are usually reinsured by the payer's own insurance.

Physician payments are also complex. When performing pretransplant donor or recipient services, such as donor evaluation or kidney excision, physicians are reimbursed through the transplant cost center for these services. It is important to recognize that nonevaluation services (ie, non–transplant-related services) to the same patient have to be charged directly to Medicare and follow the same guidelines as any part B reimbursement. A classic example would be a patient having an abdominal radiograph as part of determining eligibility for a transplant. This study and the interpretation are billed to the pretransplant cost center. If the radiograph determines the presence of a cancer and the physician schedules further evaluation and treatment of the cancer, these services are billed directly by the physician to Medicare. Once the patient completes the treatment and is sent back to complete the pretransplant evaluation, charges can again be accrued on the cost report. Posttransplant payments to physicians are not different from the usual Medicare payments for hospitalized surgical patients, with the exception that transplant surgeons can charge for postoperative immunosuppression care using specialized codes for immunosuppression management.

Having the infrastructure in the hospital and having the hospital responsible for the outcomes and holding it accountable to Medicare for the transplant program dictates the structuring of transplant programs as hospital-based programs, which is the norm in the United States (with only a few exceptions).

MANAGING THE TRANSPLANT CENTER

To achieve their goals in building successful transplantation services, hospitals have to rely on strong physician leadership and skilled administrators. Because of the dependence of transplant operations on multiple hospital departments, successful conduct of the transplant business usually requires direct high-level reporting of the transplant center administration to the highest operational leader within the organization.

The transplant business structure is also more complex than other academic departments or hospital service lines because of the multitude of reporting relationships of physicians involved in transplantation, with many having medical school appointments and positions in clinical practice organizations. This triumvirate of academic, practice, and hospital relations complicates the ability of transplant services to respond to the external environment because conflicting goals and duplicate overlapping administrative structures with subtle but distinctive differences attempt to react to service needs and to changes in reimbursement and regulatory environment.

REGULATORY COMPLIANCE IN TRANSPLANTATION

Transplantation is one of the most regulated fields in medicine.[11] This extensive regulatory oversight has evolved from the reliance of the transplantation effort on governmental resources and public trust to maintain the voluntary system of organ donation and from the expanded role of public payment for transplantation through the Medicare program.

Government oversight of transplantation started in 1984 by the National Organ Transplant Act,[12] which established a membership organization for all transplant centers and organ-procurement organizations in the United States: The Organ Procurement and Transplant Network (OPTN).[13] The OPTN has federal oversight from the Health and Human Services Administration, which, through its division of organ transplantation, oversees the OPTN contract and the contract for the Scientific Registry of Transplantation (SRTR). The Centers for Medicare and Medicaid services (CMS) started certifying transplant centers in the early 1980s and in 2007 introduced sweeping regulation that requires centers to conform to specific conditions of participation and to apply for recertification every 3 years.[14] The United Network for Organ Sharing (UNOS), which had been the sole OPTN contractor since 1986, also has oversight responsibility over organ procurement and allocation, patient listing, and data collection.[15] UNOS also defines the criteria for qualification of essential transplant personnel and reviews key personnel changes in all transplant programs for appropriateness of qualification. The data collected by UNOS on transplant outcomes are published partly by UNOS itself and by other CMS contractors, such as the SRTR.[16] Additional registries also report various transplant outcomes, such as the International Society of Heart and Lung Transplantation and the University Hospital Consortium (UHC). The data reported by the scientific registry of transplant have, over the past several years, been included in the CMS conditions of participation and used for recertification of transplant program.[14] From reported data, the SRTR calculates an expected survival for every transplant program based on the risk profile of the donors and recipients at the center. In recent years, centers not meeting the expected survival rates were required to submit corrective action plans and to undergo various audits of their clinical and administrative processes. In addition to CMS and UNOS, transplant hospitals are certified by the Joint Commission or other similar agencies and are also inspected by state authorities. Maintaining transplant certification and compliance has evolved into one of the main functions of the transplant administrators and program directors. Successful compliance requires structuring strong transplant-focused quality-improvement effort and maintaining strict policy compliance. Many public and private organizations have developed programs and consultation services to support the transplant centers in maintaining compliance. Most notable is the American Society of Transplant Surgeons that developed, through its Business Practice Committee, a continuously updated library of transplantation program policies and a consulting group that performs mock audits to prepare centers for UNOS and Medicare certification visits.

The increasing emphasis on statistical result comparisons has created a dilemma for transplant programs, forcing them to be risk averse. This risk-avoidance behavior is manifested by restricting transplantation services for higher-risk recipients, declining the use of less-than-ideal donors, and by a reluctance to attempt experimental therapies or procedures. Being risk averse limits the ability of transplant centers to serve the growing number of patients added to the waiting lists, restricts the use of potentially usable organ donors, slows advances in transplantation therapies,[17] and can potentially restrict the transplant centers' ability to grow business. This inherent tension between regulation and expansion is a major issue in building, maintaining, and expanding transplant centers.

DEFINING THE TRANSPLANTATION AND ORGAN-FAILURE BUSINESSES

A transplant center or service line differs from other traditional practices in that it integrates multiple departments, practices, and partners in order to successfully manage patient care. Defining the area of focus or mission of a transplant center is crucial to the alignment of the function of the physicians and health care providers performing the clinical functions.[18] Defining the mission of the transplant business unit is also crucial to the ability of the organization to plan for the needed resources and for the expected outcomes from the transplant effort.[19] The traditional definition of the transplant endeavor is that it is a unit that functions solely around the performance of transplants. This traditional definition limits the scope of the transplant center to immediate peritransplant activities, such as patient selection and listing, performing the actual transplant procedures, and early care of posttransplant recipients. Although powerful as a template for creating a core team of care providers, the transplant-restricted definition has multiple limitations in the evolving environment of transplantation practice, particularly as the health care system adopts a more comprehensive approach to care and progresses to new models of care, such as accountable care organizations and medical homes.[20] The first limitation is to the patients, who view the umbrella provider, usually the hospital or medical school, as a single health system and become dissatisfied by the process of internal transfer of care that inevitably occurs as they progress through their disease course to the transplant event and then to long-term care. The second limitation is related to appropriate accounting for physician revenue and hospital support to the transplant effort, both of which get complicated by the transplant-restricted mission because this restricted definition forces the organization to "silo" physician revenue into transplant-related and non–transplant-related endeavors. This artificial separation limits the organization's ability to recognize the need for supporting medical practices that are not labeled as part of the transplant service but are necessary, or even crucial, for the growth of the transplant program. This limitation has been most evident in the evolution of modern hepatology programs and in the recognition of their role as drivers for the growth of liver transplantation.[21] Similar dynamics are now evolving with heart failure cardiology and transplant and critical care pulmonology in heart and lung transplant settings. The third limitation is that the restricted transplant-focused definition of the scope of activity of the center complicates accounting for both upstream and downstream revenue[22] from transplant programs and, thus, limits the ability of an organization to fully account for the spectrum and draw of the transplant activity. This limitation could have ramifications to the provision of necessary support that can drive growth of the service line. So although a hospital can perform a small number of heart transplants and left ventricular assist devices, the availability of these services influences the pattern of referral of patients with heart failure to the hospital and distinguishes the institution from others that do not offer these treatment options. Finally, understanding the expanded scope of transplantation services is relevant considering the mechanisms for payment for these services. Having a transplantation service qualifies the hospital for financial reimbursement for the management of patients with organ failure as part of the pre-transplant evaluation services.

With these considerations, transplant centers are increasingly articulating in their mission their role in disease management and delivery of care for *patients* with organ failure.[23] This expansion of the transplant center mission to a disease management home for patients with organ failure has been one of the challenges to hospital and physician leaders, particularly in view of the increasing complexity of managing chronic diseases. Envisioning and supporting a defined transplant organization can achieve major advantages to the organization. First is that this moves beyond a model that recognizes as essential transplant providers only the physicians and surgeons essential to transplantation care. A transplant center defined around physicians and activities of caring for patients with organ failure creates a team better equipped to manage care across the continuum of the diseases that are treated by transplantation.[24] In addition, this expanded definition integrates more fully the efforts of team members to include all the physicians, departments, heath care providers, and re-searchers necessary for the growth of the organ-failure management and transplantation practice (**Fig. 1**). Integrating the care of patients with organ failure in the transplant

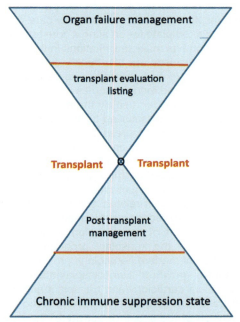

Fig. 1. Transplantation is the central point for progression of organ failure patients through phases of care. The organ-specialized physicians (hepatologists, cardiologists) perform organ-failure management and also participate in patient selection for transplantation and for pre-transplant management with transplant surgeons. The transplant phase is followed by the early posttransplant management whereby surgeons, transplant-trained organ specialists, and service-specialized physicians (pathologists, infectious diseases, rehabilitation medicine, and so forth) are key parts of the management. In lifelong management of patients, the organ-specialized physicians, endocrinologists, general internal medical physicians and others coordinate care of the patients.

center allows the organization to fully assimilate the business development, marketing, and public awareness campaigns needed to grow and sustain the center and, thus, to best serve bigger groups of its patients. Although an expanded center definition requires more complex tracking and multiple outcomes, as the notion of care evolves, this extra effort is rewarded by the improvement in the desired outcomes, both medical and financial.

THE TRANSPLANT CENTER AND SERVICE LINE

The need for remodeling transplant organizations and the creation of true transplant centers has long been articulated by transplantation thought leaders and is finally gaining momentum at various institutions.[25] The reorganization of the transplant business structure involves breaking barriers erected by traditional structures and creating new working models that improve the functionality of the team[26] in order to promote collaboration and use best practices around a focus area to drive business results.[27] This model becomes a powerful tool because its components encapsulate several key factors that, when executed together, drive up the success of a business and the attainment of its established goals. In transplantation, the definition of a team is not only a collection of staff, faculty, and administrators but also invokes the idea of teamwork.[28] Also, implicit in the definition is the alignment of resource, time expenditure, costs, and profits to the business unit or service line. The success of a transplant center, therefore, requires not only the careful creation of a winning team but also the explicit definition of the focus area, an understanding of the desired goals, and a developed rubric for scoring success. The necessity of predefining these metrics becomes evident in the value a transplant center adds to its organization.

UNDERSTANDING AND BENCHMARKING THE TRANSPLANT BUSINESS

One of the main needs for any business or business organization is to understand their customer and their customers' needs. Potential customers of a transplant center include the patients, the payers, and the referring physicians. Internal customers, just as important to the survival of a transplant center, include transplant center and hospital staff. Without considering these internal customers and attempting to truly serve them, the transplant center will be plagued by low patient satisfaction, high turnover, and potentially catastrophic near misses and process breakdowns. Success in meeting the needs of each customer group must have its own metric, that is, clinical measures for patients, process measures for internal staff, contract execution for payers, and a referral pattern for referring physicians (**Fig. 2**). Identifying who is served by the transplant center lies at the heart of the development of the endeavor. The task of understanding how to deliver value to these various customers will drive the enterprise performance success metrics.[29]

PATIENT-CENTERED OUTCOMES

It is imperative that a transplant center, as a patient-focused enterprise, has a set of clinical patient-centered outcomes at the core of its scorecard.[30] The results can be assessed by comparing outcomes with expected norms such as those published by the SRTR or the UHC or with other benchmarks that are developed locally in areas where no published measures exist.[31] Monitoring and measuring success in the organ-failure management portion of the transplant business can be complex but is now facilitated by identifying the relevant DRGs associated with the nontransplant

Balanced score card
Transplant center

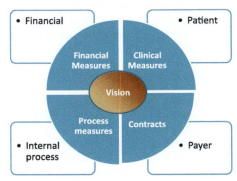

Fig. 2. Monitoring progress in a transplant center of excellence: Create a balanced scorecard that is based on the center's vision and mission and monitors the outcomes of the processes and the primary customers of the center.

episodes of care. These DRGs can be used to compare performance with national benchmarks such as those published by the UHC or with community-based benchmarks available through the American Hospital Association (AHA) or other similar organizations.

Transplant volume has been traditionally used as a measure for growth and infrastructure support for transplant centers.[32] Justifying the use of the transplant volume in this fashion is the fact that volume is a proxy for the episodes of care associated with the greatest financial contribution to the hospital bottom line. The volumes of preoperative and postoperative episodes of care are also crucial to measure and track because they underscore the need for resources beyond the in-hospital transplant phase (**Table 1**). Implied in the utilization volumes of care episodes as a benchmark is the realization of the need to sensitively monitor expansion in all aspects of patient

Table 1
Benchmarking resource needs in a transplant center

Patient Contact	Low	Moderate	High	Total
Heart	2457	1103	152	3712
Lung	2293	357	51	2701
Kidney	11,654	2395	270	14,319
Liver	4855	498	99	5452
Pancreas	665	162	15	842

Patient visits are divided by number, intensity, and duration. The definition of high-intensity visit includes one with complex medical issues, extensive counseling and education, and follow-up by coordinator or physician contact. Low-intensity contacts include visits with routine medical problems and/or standard testing review. These data are used to assign a mixture of patient contacts to each coordinator and coordinator assistant and to make projections from the volume regarding the future needs of the program.

Data from Houston Methodist J.C. Walter Transplant Center Planning Document with 2009 data-Methodology based on: Flood SD, Diers D. Nurse staffing, patient outcome and cost. Nurs Manager 1988;19(5):34–5, 38–9, 42–3.

interactions to increase productivity and the realization that these episodes can generate a positive bottom line either independently or through creating more transplants. Adequate funding of these activities is by far the most important determinant of growth in transplant volumes over time. Lastly, clinical profitability measures are important to track, in some form, by the center leadership. Proxies for clinical profitability, such as length of hospital stay, readmissions, and return to the operating room, are popular to track and correlate well with overall profitability. These clinical-benchmarks also identify to the clinical leadership the need for evidence-based process development - as they underscore the positive impact of quality improvement on clinical and financial performance. Because of the complexity of reimbursements and contracts, clinical proxies should not substitute for tracking real-time financial benchmarks, such as average charge, cost, and reimbursement per transplant. Importantly, tracking financial performance and understanding the simple concepts of fixed and variable costs and their relationship to the contribution margin and profitability are important to focus the efforts of the center leadership on outcome-based cost control. Creating a balanced scorecard that tracks all of these outcomes simultaneously allows the medical and administrative leadership to make decisions based on an understanding of the overall position of the enterprise.

Finally, because physician leadership plays a crucial role in transplant center management and success,[33] a transplant center charter should create monitors of leadership performance that track the success of the leaders in the creation of a positive organizational culture that stresses transparency, execution, and the satisfaction of all primary customers.

REFERENCES

1. Childress JF. The gift of life: ethical problems and policies in obtaining and distributing organs for transplantation. Prim Care 1986;13(2):379-94.
2. Caplan AL. Requests, gifts, and obligations: the ethics of organ procurement. Transplant Proc 1986;18(3 Suppl 2):49-56.
3. Rosner F, Henry JB, Wolpaw JR, et al. Ethical and social issues in organ procurement for transplantation. N Y State J Med 1993;93:30-4.
4. Herring AA, Woolhandler S, Himmelstein DU. Insurance status of U.S. organ donors and transplant recipients: the uninsured give, but rarely receive. Transplantation 1992;53(5):1041-6.
5. Evans RW. Public and private insurer designation of transplantation programs. Transplantation 1992;5(5):1041-6.
6. Beach-Langlois M, Yankasky P. Transplant cost-report tracking at Henry Ford Transplant Institute and other centers nationwide. Prog Transplant 2011;21(2):169-73.
7. Abecassis M. Organ acquisition cost centers part I: Medicare regulations-truth or consequence. Am J Transplant 2006;6(12):2830-5.
8. Englesbe MJ, Dimick JB, Fan Z, et al. Case mix, quality and high-cost kidney transplant patients. Am J Transplant 2009;9(5):1108-14.
9. Marshall B, Swearingen JP. Complexities in transplant revenue management. Prog Transplant 2007;17(2):94-8.
10. Keough CL. CMS establishes new audit requirements, proposes new overpayment rule. Healthc Financ Manage 2002;56(4):92-4.
11. Festle MJ. Enemies or allies? The organ transplant medical community, the federal government, and the public in the United States, 1967-2000. J Hist Med Allied Sci 2010;65(1):48-80.

12. Blumstein JF. Government's role in organ transplantation policy [review]. J Health Polit Policy Law 1989;14(1):5–39.
13. Medicare and Medicaid programs; organ procurement and transplantation network rules and membership actions–HCFA. General notice. Fed Regist 1989;54(241):51802–3.
14. Available at: http://www.cms.gov/Medicare/Provider-Enrollment-and-Certification/CertificationandComplianc/Transplant.html. Accessed October 1, 2013.
15. Brown RS Jr, Higgins R, Pruett TL. The evolution and direction of OPTN oversight of live organ donation and transplantation in the United States. Am J Transplant 2009;9(1):31–4.
16. Leppke S, Leighton T, Zaun D, et al. Scientific registry of transplant recipients: collecting, analyzing, and reporting data on transplantation in the United States. Transplant Rev (Orlando) 2013;27(2):50–6.
17. Abecassis MM, Burke R, Cosimi AB, et al. Transplant center regulations–a mixed blessing? An ASTS Council viewpoint; American Society of Transplant Surgeons. Am J Transplant 2008;8(12):2496–502.
18. Kaplan RS, Norton DP. Mastering the management system. Harv Bus Rev 2008; 86:62–77, 136.
19. Sloan TB, Kaye CI, Allen WR, et al. Implementing a simpler approach to mission-based planning in a medical school. Acad Med 2005;80:994–1004.
20. Axelrod DA, Millman D, Abecassis MM. US health care reform and transplantation, part II: impact on the public sector and novel health care delivery systems. Am J Transplant 2010;10(10):2203.
21. Shiffman ML, Rockey DC. Role and support for hepatologists at lover transplant programs in the United States. Liver Transpl 2008;14:1092–109.
22. Cohen SM, Gundlapalli S, Shah AR, et al. The downstream financial effect of hepatology. Hepatology 2005;41:968–75.
23. Wigg AJ, McCormick R, Wundke R, et al. Efficacy of a chronic disease management model for patients with chronic liver failure. Clin Gastroenterol Hepatol 2013; 11(7):850–8.e1-4.
24. Ofman JJ, Badamgarav E, Henning JM, et al. Does disease management improve clinical and economic outcomes in patients with chronic diseases? A systematic review. Am J Med 2004;117:182–92.
25. Howard RJ, Kaplan B. The time is now: formation of true transplant centers. Am J Transplant 2008;8:2225–9.
26. Turnipseed WD, Lund DP, Sollenberger D. Product line development: a strategy for clinical success in academic centers. Ann Surg 2007;246:585–90 [discussion: 590–2].
27. Strickler J. What is a center of excellence. AgileElements. 2008. Available at: http://agileelements.wordpress.com/2008/10/29/what-is-a-center-of-excellence/. Accessed October 1, 2013.
28. Gratton L, Erickson TJ. 8 ways to build collaborative teams. Harv Bus Rev 2007; 85:100–9, 153.
29. Longshore GF. Service in-line management/bottom-line management. J Health Care Finance 1998;24:72–9.
30. Randolph G, Esporas M, Provost L, et al. Model for improvement – part two: measurement and feedback for quality improvement efforts. Pediatr Clin North Am 2009;56:779–98.
31. Axelrod DA, Guidinger MK, Metzger RA, et al. Transplant center quality assessment using a continuously updatable, risk-adjusted technique (CUSUM). Am J Transplant 2006;6:313–23.

32. Axelrod DA, Guidinger MK, McCullough KP, et al. Association of center volume with outcome after liver and kidney transplantation. Am J Transplant 2004;4: 920–7.
33. Schwartz RW, Pogge C. Physician leadership: essential skills in a changing environment. Am J Surg 2000;180:187–92.

Index

Note: Page numbers of article titles are in **boldface** type.

A

Adenoma(s)
  liver
    HCC due to, 1426
Aflatoxin
  HCC due to, 1426
Age
  as factor in robotic-assisted kidney transplantation, 1311
Alcohol injection
  in HCC management, 1435
Alcoholic cirrhosis
  HCC due to, 1425
AMR. *See* Antibody-mediated rejection (AMR)
Anesthesia/anesthetics
  in left lobe liver transplantation, 1330
Antibody-mediated rejection (AMR)
  classification of, 1452–1453
  diagnosis of, 1452–1453
  in transplantation, **1451–1466**
    management of, **1451–1466**
      antibody removal in, 1453–1454
      B-cell–specific agents in, 1454–1456
      bortezomib in, 1456–1458
      chronic, 1462
      complement-specific agents in, 1458–1459
      future clinical trials in, 1462
      introduction, 1451–1452
      IVIg in, 1454
      plasma cell–depleting agents in, 1456–1458
      rituximab in, 1454–1456
      splenectomy in, 1459–1462
Antibody removal
  in AMR management, 1453–1454
Anticoagulation
  LVADs and, 1351–1354
Antimetabolic agents
  in renal transplantation, 1299
Aspiration
  EVLP in management of, 1386–1387

Surg Clin N Am 93 (2013) 1479–1489
http://dx.doi.org/10.1016/S0039-6109(13)00172-2
0039-6109/13/$ – see front matter © 2013 Elsevier Inc. All rights reserved.

surgical.theclinics.com

Index page.

Moving?

Make sure your subscription moves with you!

To notify us of your new address, find your **Clinics Account Number** (located on your mailing label above your name), and contact customer service at:

Email: journalscustomerservice-usa@elsevier.com

800-654-2452 (subscribers in the U.S. & Canada)
314-447-8871 (subscribers outside of the U.S. & Canada)

Fax number: 314-447-8029

Elsevier Health Sciences Division
Subscription Customer Service
3251 Riverport Lane
Maryland Heights, MO 63043

Printed and bound by CPI Group (UK) Ltd, Croydon, CR0 4YY

08/06/2025

01896870-0001